SWEET POISON

DAVID GILLESPIE is a recovering corporate lawyer, co-founder of a successful software company and consultant to the IT industry. He is also a father of six young children (including one set of twins). With such a lot of extra time on his hands, and 40 extra kilos on his waistline, he set out to investigate why he, like so many in his generation, was fat. He deciphered the latest medical findings on diet and weight gain and what he found was chilling. Being fat was the least of his problems. He needed to stop poisoning himself.

David is also the author of the bestselling *The Sweet Poison Quit Plan* and *Big Fat Lies*. Find out more at sweetpoison.com.au.

Praise for *Sweet Poison*

'What's impressive about *Sweet Poison* is that Gillespie turns complex research on what happens to food inside our body and its relation to weight gain into a good read.'
Sydney Morning Herald

'Comprehensive, thought provoking and highly readable.'
The Age

'Eye-opening.'
Woman's Day

'David Gillespie's groundbreaking book on the dangers of a high sugar intake could well revolutionise the way you diet.'
A Current Affair

'*Sweet Poison* is a worthy and impassioned effort by an Australian dad to share his surprising discoveries with struggling dieters and provoke further debate about the obesity epidemic.'
Australian Bookseller & Publisher

'This is a life-changing book. I wish I'd read it 25 years ago, but now I'm 25 kilos lighter – simply by understanding and embracing the basic principles in *Sweet Poison*.'
Peter FitzSimons

'I've lost 11kg without being on a diet.
It's good to know this book is non-fiction.'
Steve Irons MP, Member of the Parliamentary Inquiry into Obesity

SWEET POISON

WHY SUGAR MAKES US FAT

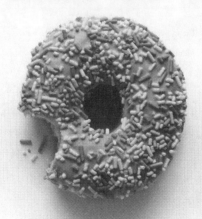

DAVID GILLESPIE

VIKING

an imprint of

PENGUIN BOOKS

For Lizzie, Anthony, James,
Gwendolen, Adam, Elizabeth and Finlayson.

VIKING

Published by the Penguin Group
Penguin Group (Australia)
707 Collins Street, Melbourne 3008, Victoria, Australia
(a division of Pearson Australia Group Pty Ltd)
Penguin Group (USA) Inc.
375 Hudson Street, New York, New York 10014, USA
Penguin Group (Canada)
90 Eglinton Avenue East, Suite 700, Toronto, Canada ON M4P 2Y3
(a division of Pearson Penguin Canada Inc.)
Penguin Books Ltd
80 Strand, London WC2R 0RL England
Penguin Ireland
25 St Stephen's Green, Dublin 2, Ireland
(a division of Penguin Books Ltd)
Penguin Books India Pvt Ltd
11 Community Centre, Panchsheel Park, New Delhi – 110 017, India
Penguin Group (NZ)
67 Apollo Drive, Rosedale, North Shore 0632, New Zealand
(a division of Pearson New Zealand Ltd)
Penguin Books (South Africa) (Pty) Ltd
24 Sturdee Avenue, Rosebank, Johannesburg 2196, South Africa

Penguin Books Ltd, Registered Offices: 80 Strand, London, WC2R 0RL, England

First published by Penguin Group (Australia), 2008

19 20

Copyright © David Gillespie 2008

The moral right of the author has been asserted

Cover design by Daniel New © Penguin Group (Australia)
Text design by Kirby Stalgis © Penguin Group (Australia)
Cover photograph by Getty Images
Typeset in 11.5/17 pt Berkeley Oldstyle by Post Pre-press Group, Brisbane, Queensland
Printed and bound in Australia by McPherson's Printing Group, Maryborough, Victoria

National Library of Australia
Cataloguing-in-Publication data:

Gillespie, David, 1966–
Sweet poison / David Gillespie.
1st ed.
978 067 007247 7 (pbk.).
Sugar – Health aspects.
Food – Sugar content.

613.283

penguin.com.au

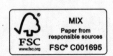

Contents

Introduction

I still remember the day Lizzie told me. She had a stunned, almost fearful expression on her face and was unsure of herself in a way I had rarely seen in my wife of 13 years. Our fifth and assumedly last child had just been turned into twins with a wave of the ultrasound wand. In about eight months, we were to become parents of six children under nine years of age. I was about 40kg overweight, and had struggled with my weight for as long as I could remember (except for a brief period during university when I managed to snare Lizzie). I had tried most things, from reducing fat in my diet to not eating to regularly attending the gym and walking the dog. Sometimes I had had limited success (a few kilograms here and there), but it was mostly small backward steps on my ever-accelerating journey to obesity and beyond.

With the weight came lethargy and sleeping problems. As any parent could attest, getting enough sleep and having the energy to get through the day is difficult at the best of times, let alone when you're starting out in the red. I was going to have to be a dad to twin babies and four other young children and I couldn't see myself managing it carrying 40 extra kilos, feeling lethargic and not sleeping.

At the time, the Atkins diet was beginning to take off, with all manner of people touting it as a miracle diet. My uncle had recently undergone heart surgery and was now on Atkins. He had lost a vast amount of weight and was tucking into bacon and eggs every morning for breakfast. This looked like a diet I could really enjoy. I immediately cut out all carbs and, lo and behold, I started losing weight like never before (although I suspect it was because I found it almost impossible to find any food I wanted to eat that did not contain carbohydrates). I spent a couple of weeks feeling like I was starving to death. The weight was coming off but the willpower required to stay on the diet was overwhelming (not to mention the nasty side effects that eliminating fibre from my diet was having). I started to look for alternatives. At first low-GI diets seemed appealing, because they at least allowed you to eat some carbohydrates, but almost no foods were labelled with GI indicators and the maths involved in calculating it myself was beyond me. When chocolate spreads advertised their low-GI levels, I knew that if a food that was half sugar and half fat could earn a low-GI label, the GI calculation was probably almost meaningless for dieters.

I had been reading a lot about Charles Darwin's life and his works on evolution. Darwin's theories held that all characteristics of modern animals were survival responses developed slowly over millennia. As a result, we (and all animals) are woefully inadequate at dealing with sudden changes in the environment. After reading about these theories, it had occurred to me that my weight gain, and that of most other people in our society, could not possibly be down to a lack of willpower alone (since willpower, or the lack of it, would be an evolved characteristic that could not suddenly have changed in just a few hundred years). In a desperate attempt to find a way to keep up the weight loss without having to stay on the carb-free diet, I started to read up on human metabolism. I quickly came to the conclusion that I would have to learn a whole new vocabulary to understand most of what was being written. However, I was beginning to get the vague feeling that many in the medical profession took for granted a fact that was a complete mystery to the rest of us.

Study after study seemed to be pointing to the inescapable conclusion that the fructose part of sugar was fat-inducing in animals, and probably in humans as well. Worse still, it seemed to be complicit in making us want to eat more food in general. Although I found many studies within the medical fraternity backing this line of thought, documents written for the rest of us were almost impossible to find. Those that did exist were, more often than not, rants against sugar in general without any explanation as to why it was bad for us. I immediately changed from eliminating carbs to just eliminating foods with added sugar – at last I could eat bread again. It was impossible to remove all sugar because everything seems to contain it, so I set myself a limit of no more than 10g of sugar in a meal (about the amount of fructose in an apple). This simply meant I no longer ate sweets and biscuits or drank juice and soft drink. The weight loss continued, but the diet was a lot easier to stick to. After a few months, I was so used to not having sugar that it took no willpower at all to refuse it. In fact, on the few occasions I did try chocolates, they tasted unbearably sweet.

I've now lost the 40kg and, more importantly, no longer worry about weight gain at all. I know that I can eat when I feel hungry and stop eating when I feel full and I will not put on weight. I can eat whatever I like whenever I feel like eating, as long as it does not include sugar. I have no urge to eat when I'm not hungry, I no longer feel lethargic or sleep deprived (other than as would be expected for a father of six), and no unnecessary exercise was involved at all. By far the greatest benefit has been the ability to trust my own body to let me know when to eat and when not to. It's a feeling I've never experienced before.

People obviously noticed the change in my appearance and energy levels, and asked me what I had done. 'I stopped eating sugar' seemed too trite and forwarding them medical journal articles just a little bit over the top, so I decided the story of the sweet poison had to be written in language we all could understand.

PART 1
WHY IS SUGAR MAKING YOU FAT?

1. STARTING OUT

One of the first articles I came across during my 'net-education' was a book written over 40 years ago with the catchy title *The Saccharine Disease*. This quaintly written 129-page book, authored by Surgeon-Captain Cleave of Her Majesty's Navy in 1966, caught my eye because it contained a theory that there was a strong link between evolution and diet. This matched up with some of the thoughts I had been having after reading about Charles Darwin's theories on evolution.

The good doctor was saying that the human body, having evolved in an environment of a largely wholegrain, vegetable and (occasional) meat diet, was ill-equipped to deal with the highly processed sugar and refined flour diet of the twentieth century. Dr Cleave had decided, after a lifetime of treating sick sailors (he was 60 when he wrote the book), that a huge number of modern diseases were directly caused by the over-consumption of sugar and refined flour. He blamed sugar and flour for the headline diseases like obesity, coronary disease and diabetes. But he also threw in peptic ulcer, constipation, haemorrhoids and varicose veins, as well as appendicitis, gallstones, urinary tract infection, inflammation of the large intestine and, of course, dental cavities, among others.

This book was clearly written with a medically trained audience in mind, so I don't recommend it for a relaxing read in front of the fire. I'm certainly no doctor and I came across this book at the very beginning of my reading, so most of its analysis went straight over my head. There was, however, one graph – that's right, I went straight for the pictures – that really got me interested in the theory behind Dr Cleave's 'saccharine disease'. Chapter 2 contained a graph that showed that sugar consumption in England had risen eightfold between 1815 and 1955. The average inhabitant of the British Isles was consuming just 15lb (about 7kg) of sugar in 1817. By 1955, their intake was almost 110lb (50kg). The steady upward march had only been briefly interrupted by the intervention of the two world wars.

The Surgeon-Captain was convinced that this rise in sugar consumption, along with a similar trend in the consumption of refined white flour, was entirely responsible for the raft of illnesses that he collectively dubbed 'the saccharine disease'. Dr Cleave had noticed that all of the diseases he was including were virtually nonexistent prior to 1900 and he simply put two and two together. The diseases were increasing at about the same rate as the consumption of sugar and refined flour. According to him, it was the concentration (by refinement) that was the problem with both sugar and flour. When sugar is refined from cane or sugar beet, 99 per cent of the original food (mostly the fibre) is removed, leaving only the sugar syrup. Similarly, by the time white flour is created, 90 per cent of the bran has been removed. The thinking was that by removing the fibre, we were making food much easier to digest. Sugar and flour would be reduced to glucose by the body and, without the fibre to slow things down, the glucose would hit our bloodstream very quickly. Dr Cleave felt this would 'upset the evolutionary adaptation in the pancreas [where it] is held . . . to cause the disease'.

The solution was obvious to Cleave. Just add bran to everything you eat. Legend has it that while serving as the ship's doctor aboard the battleship *King George V* during World War II, he would have large sacks of bran brought on board to 'prescribe' to the crew. I think he could have counted himself lucky that the worst nickname he acquired as a result was 'the bran man'.

I was intrigued by the enormous growth in sugar consumption shown in the graph. Sugar consumption was clearly growing at an extraordinary rate and some of Dr Cleave's other graphs showed that diabetes and other diseases were growing at similar rates. But I was less convinced by his argument that adding bran to your diet to counteract the excess sugar and flour was the secret to avoiding so many diseases. I needed to understand more about the chemistry involved in digestion before I was prepared to start pouring bran on my chocolate ice-cream. This, unfortunately, would involve my getting very close to some subjects that I had avoided since I almost failed Biology and Chemistry in high school. But I am one of those people who can't leave a problem alone until I am convinced I have worked out a logically consistent argument for how the whole system works. And Dr Cleave's clogged-up pancreas wasn't doing it for me.

By the time you get to the end of this book, you'll figure out (as I did) that Dr Cleave wasn't too far from the mark. All right, it's called 'metabolic syndrome' rather than 'the saccharine disease', and it's a part of sugar that's the problem, not refined flour and sugar. But the pancreas does play a role and fibre is part of the prevention. He got close to the right answer from his observations, but (as with most things in life) the details were significantly more complex than I am sure he ever imagined.

There is no shortage of 'educational' resources about human digestion on the internet. After reading a few of the more 'interesting' theories about digestion and how it works, I decided to stick to sites that doctors seemed to regard as authoritative: mostly medical journals, or sites run by people who publish articles in medical journals. Unfortunately, all of these articles appeared to have been written on the presumption that I had completed six years of medical school and practised gastroenterology (the study of the human digestive system) and endocrinology (the study of the human hormone-producing organs) for at least 20 years. I had a steep learning curve ahead of me and it took me a long time to get up to speed, looking up every second word on Wikipedia along the way. I won't bore you with the detail of all the false starts and blind alleys, but here is what I discovered (in English rather than Latin and Greek).

The sugar that Dr Cleave was talking about is common table sugar, the white (or brown) stuff some of us add to our cup of tea in the morning to make it a bit more pleasurable to drink. It's the same sugar that, in Australia and the United Kingdom, is added to most foods that require sweetening. In the United States they use a cheaper substance called high-fructose corn syrup (HFCS) for sweetening processed food. HFCS is, for all practical purposes, identical to sugar, despite what some of the more excitable websites would have you believe. But more on that later . . .

It seems cocoa, tea and coffee merchants were in fact almost single-handedly responsible for introducing sugar into the English (and hence the western) diet. As anyone who has tried even '80 per cent cocoa' dark chocolate will attest, cocoa is a pretty bitter pill to swallow without sugar. But add some of the sweet stuff and suddenly you have a product that flies off the shelves. The same goes for tea and coffee, so the only way the merchants bringing these new foods into the western world could convince people to drink their newly introduced bitter beverages in the sixteenth century was to suggest the addition of the newly discovered sweetener, cane sugar.

Sometimes it's called caster sugar or raw sugar or brown sugar or white sugar, but it's all the same stuff. It's what most of us think of when asked to describe sugar. Scientists call table sugar (and all its variants) 'sucrose'. The group of compounds with chemical properties like table sugar are generically called 'sugars' by chemists and nutritionists. This makes it all pretty confusing since what ordinary people call sugar and what scientists and nutritionists call sugar are in fact two different (but overlapping) things.

Sucrose (table sugar) is a double sugar (disaccharide – Latin for two sugars). This simply means that it is made up of two 'simple sugars' – glucose and fructose – joined together at the molecular level. Just as this is starting to sound confusing, it turns out that our digestive system doesn't bother remembering complex names either. To your digestive system there is no such thing as sucrose. When you eat a teaspoon (5g) of sucrose, your body 'sees' 2.5g of glucose and 2.5g of fructose.

There are only three important simple sugars: glucose, fructose and galactose. All of the other 'sugars' you are likely to encounter in daily life are simply combinations of these three. For example, the 'sugar' you see on the label of a carton of milk is lactose. Lactose is half glucose and half galactose. Maltose, the sugar in beer, is two molecules of glucose joined together in an unusual way.

Simple sugars like glucose and fructose can also be present in nature in their uncombined form. Most fruit, for example, contains some sucrose, some fructose and some glucose. To our digestive system, however, the sucrose is just a bundle of more fructose and glucose.

This food . . .	Contains . . .	Which breaks down to . . .
Milk and dairy foods	Lactose	Galactose + glucose
Beer	Maltose	Glucose + glucose
Table sugar, brown sugar, caster sugar, etc.	Sucrose	Glucose + fructose

Figure 1.1: All those different 'oses' break down to one of three important sugars.

Glucose is by far the most plentiful of the simple sugars. Pretty much every food (except meat) contains significant quantities of glucose. Even meat (protein) is eventually converted to glucose by our digestive system. It's a pretty important sugar to humans. Pure glucose tastes slightly sweet, but would be barely noticeable to the sugar-saturated palate of the modern human. Australian readers who have recently been to the pharmacist will insist this is not true, citing a brand of jelly bean stocked only by chemists as evidence to the contrary. Unfortunately, a quick look at the label reveals that the primary ingredient is in fact sugar. The sweetness comes from the fructose part of the molecule.

Galactose is present in our environment in only very small quantities and is found mainly in dairy products in the form of lactose. Most baby mammals, including humans, are adapted to survive on lactose when they are young, but about 70 per cent of the world's adult human population are lactose intolerant and cannot digest lactose or use it for energy production. People with ancestry in northern Europe, the Middle East and India (the places where people have the longest association with domesticated cattle), however, have a version of the lactose digestion gene that is not disabled when they grow up. Those people (most of the Australian population) are able to continue to drink and eat milk products comfortably into adulthood. Those of us who can digest galactose convert it to glucose and treat it as glucose for all important digestive purposes. Everybody else lets it pass straight through the digestive system, which is why a primary symptom of lactose intolerance is diarrhoea. Galactose is slightly less sweet than glucose, but it's still on the sweet side of the palate. If you are not lactose intolerant, pay close attention to the next glass of milk you consume. You will notice an ever so slight sweet tinge to the flavour – it is certainly not sour (at least if you drink it before the use-by date).

Fructose is also relatively rare in nature. It is found primarily in ripe fruits, which is why it is sometimes call fruit sugar. It is usually found together with glucose and sometimes sucrose. Fructose tastes about 60 per cent sweeter than glucose or galactose. In practical terms this means you would need to consume 2 teaspoons of glucose to get the same sweetness hit that you would from 1 teaspoon of fructose. Table sugar, being a combination of the two, is halfway between in terms of sweetness. As with lactose, consumption of a large amount of pure fructose can result in exceeding the capacity of our intestines to absorb it, resulting in diarrhoea. If, however, fructose is eaten in combination with glucose, for example by eating sugar, then it seems we can absorb virtually unlimited quantities (more on this later).

These three 'sugars' make up the vast majority of the food group we call carbohydrates (they are made up of *carbo*n, *hydro*gen and oxygen – the 'ate' in carbohydrate indicates the presence of oxygen). The only other significant carbohydrate is cellulose, or what we commonly call fibre (the hard stringy bits of plants). If you've ever eaten a lot of baked beans in a sitting, you'll know that humans can't fully digest fibre. And over-consumption leads to exactly the same result as when a lactose-intolerant person eats too much dairy food – diarrhoea and flatulence. This doesn't mean fibre has no purpose in our digestive system; it's just that we don't use it for energy.

Only about half the western diet is carbohydrate based. In a normal diet, a further one-sixth of our energy needs are supplied by protein (predominantly from meat, but also from nuts). Protein is broken down into amino acids by our digestive system, some of which are used to build up our tissues and some to assist in hormone production. Leftover amino acids are converted to glucose and used for energy in exactly the same manner as with carbohydrate digestion. The remaining third of our food is fat. Fat is broken down into fatty acids by our digestive system. Most fatty acids are used to make all the chemicals we use to digest everything else, and some are used for energy.

This food . . .	Contains (mostly) . . .	Which breaks down to . . .
Bread	Carbohydrate	Glucose + fibre
Milk	Carbohydrate + fat	Glucose + galactose + fatty acids
Meat (or nuts)	Protein + fat	Glucose + amino acids + fatty acids
Fruit	Carbohydrate	Glucose + fructose + fibre
Vegetables	Carbohydrate	Glucose + fibre

Figure 1.2: The whole world looks like glucose to our digestive system.

If you think of your body as being like an automobile (mine started out as a minibus), then think of it as being designed to run on a fuel of pure glucose. Our preferred source is carbohydrates, which can be broken down easily into glucose, but we have some well-designed coping mechanisms to convert other foods to glucose as well.

As far as our body is concerned, everything we eat is just glucose in disguise; sometimes it's wrapped in a bit of fat or a bit of fibre, sometimes with some 'additives' (vitamins) that we can use for running repairs and maintenance, but in the end it's really just glucose. Most carbohydrates are broken down into glucose, with a few throwaway molecules of fructose and galactose. Even the galactose is either converted to glucose or expelled from the body. Protein is similarly largely reduced to glucose before being used as fuel.

Most experts seem to agree that we have existed as a separate species for about 130 000 years. This makes our current urban environment and diet (which even with the most optimistic definition has existed for only the last 10 000 years) almost completely irrelevant in determining the evolved characteristics of our digestive system. We are probably genetically identical to the people who first settled in villages in the Niger delta. And 120 000 years before that, as our forebears started roaming the African savanna, they had to select things that would provide them with energy from the available food sources and at the same time avoid things that could poison them. People who couldn't tell the difference generally didn't last long enough to reproduce. Our distant forebears had evolved a handy little energy detector. Food that contains glucose tastes slightly sweet to us so, in nature, that taste we describe as sweetness is generally a reliable indicator of the presence of an edible high-energy food. Our forebears learned that the sweeter the food, the more energy it was likely to contain. Millennia of evolution have ensured that we are programmed to seek out sweet sources of food and reject sour substances as being probably poisonous or at least to be treated with caution (meaning wait for your neighbour to give it a go first).

For all but the last few hundred years (a heartbeat on the genetic evolution time scale), really sweet foods have been difficult to find. The sweetest food we encountered in nature, fruit, had been an occasional and, depending on where you lived, relatively rare bonus in our diet. The only other way to get a sugar hit in nature involved discussing the matter with a large swarm of disgruntled bees. Honey is 40 per cent fructose, which is why, even despite the difficulty in obtaining it, it was very popular as a food additive before the discovery of sugar.

Once we figured out, towards the end of the nineteenth century, how to make any food artificially sweet by adding sugar, sugar became a pretty popular 'condiment', as the good Dr Cleave's graph clearly showed. Food manufacturers were happy to accommodate our preference for sweet foods as soon as it became commercially viable to produce sugar in large quantities. But more on the commercial side of things later – back to biology . . .

As far as I could tell, there was nothing controversial in any of the processes I have described above. How food is broken down and what supplies us with energy seems well settled (if somewhat opaquely explained by most sources). Understanding that all food is essentially glucose was an important foundation for me. (Why doesn't anybody tell us this in school? Maybe they did and I just wasn't listening.) But I hadn't figured out how the pancreas was involved (or even what the pancreas was) and why Dr Cleave would think that sugar consumption would clog it up, with all sorts of disastrous consequences. Or, for that matter, why putting bran on my food would fix it. Clearly further research was required.

2. THEORIES OF FATNESS

Most of us don't eat constantly during the day (unless we are on the 'Elvis in the '70s' diet), so our fuel intake is a bit 'lumpy'. Three times a day we take in a lot of fuel, which is just about enough to get us to the next meal. Our body, however, needs a constant fuel supply that doesn't change much over time. Life would be pretty strange if we got peak performance out of our brain, heart and kidneys only directly after a meal, with performance falling off until we were virtually comatose just before the next meal came around. It would be like having a car that only worked well just after you filled its tank.

To ensure the amount of glucose in our blood (the fuel mix, if you like) remains constant, our body uses a simple negative feedback system. When we eat, our blood-glucose levels increase as the food is broken down into its component molecules and absorbed into our bloodstream. And it seems this is where the pancreas comes in. The pancreas (from Greek, meaning 'all flesh', because it looks like a fleshy lump – but then again what organ doesn't?) is a small organ, about 15 to 25cm long in most of us, tucked in just below and behind the stomach. Older readers will know lamb and calf pancreas by the butcher's description of 'sweetbreads' (which made it a little more saleable than 'pancreas' and definitely more saleable than 'fleshy lump', I suspect). Younger readers will have no clue what I'm talking about. We are all now too affluent to bother eating offal (unless we frequent all-you-can-eat establishments where it is presented in gravy or those really fancy restaurants that are trying to make offal trendy again).

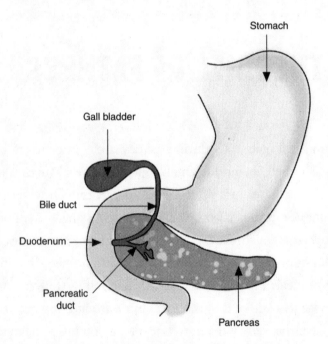

Figure 2.1: The pancreas and its neighbouring organs – not pretty, but then very little below skin level in a human is.

This fairly important piece of offal performs two basic functions for us. It produces the enzymes (proteins that accelerate chemical reactions) that break down our food into its component parts by separating the molecules.

To keep the number of names we have to remember to a minimum, the name of the enzyme that breaks down a given sugar has the same start to the sugar's name but ends in 'ase'. For example, the enzyme that breaks down lactose into glucose and galactose is called lactase. If you are lactose intolerant, your pancreas can't produce lact*ase*. This means you are unable to extract any energy from the lact*ose* and so it passes through the stomach to the intestine unmolested by enzymes. If we don't have the right enzyme, we can't digest any carbohydrate other than pure glucose, so enzymes are pretty crucial to the whole process.

Besides making the garden shears used to chemically chop up our food, the pancreas also produces the hormones that control the amount of glucose in our bloodstream – the equivalent of the throttle in my car analogy. Specialist cells in our pancreas called the islets of Langerhans monitor blood-glucose levels. These cells were named after the German biologist Paul Langerhans, who first described them in 1869 as islands of clear cells in the pancreas. Paul didn't know what they were for, but the island description stuck and so did his name.

One of the critically important hormones manufactured by the islets of Langerhans is insulin (*insula* is Latin for 'island'). Insulin is a powerful hormone that regulates many processes in the digestive system, but its primary function is to reduce glucose concentrations in our blood. The first and most obvious way to do this is to use the glucose as fuel. Most cells in our bodies use glucose as the main source of energy, but without insulin also present in the blood, the cells have no chemical means of accessing the energy stored in glucose. Insulin acts as a chemical enabler that allows the cells to absorb and then convert the glucose to energy. The only significant exception is our brain. Neurons (the cells that make up our grey matter) do not need insulin – they can suck up the glucose and use it directly from the bloodstream.

Some people need to inject insulin after a meal because their pancreas is unable to make its own. About one in every 50 000 people is unable to make insulin because their islets of Langerhans have been destroyed by their own immune system. People who study these things for a living don't know why these (usually) young bodies have destroyed their own capacity to produce such a critical hormone; however, a popular theory is that it is the result of a viral infection in childhood. These people are referred to medically as suffering from insulin-dependent diabetes, also called type 1 diabetes. This type of diabetes is really just chronic high blood sugar. For those who like impressing friends with big Greek medical words, the technical term is hyperglycaemia (*hyper* – excessive; *glyc* – sweet; and *aemia* – related to the blood).

When a person with diabetes eats, the blood fills with glucose, but without insulin present to enable its conversion to energy (or fat, as we shall see later), and because the only major organ able to use the glucose without insulin is the brain, the body maintains a state of very high blood sugar.

If you have untreated type 1 diabetes, you are not expected to have a very long or pleasant life. With most cells having no way to access the glucose in your blood, it's the medical equivalent of dying of thirst in the middle of the ocean. The body would be in a constant energy crisis because no matter what you ate, you would be unable to convert most of the glucose from the food into energy. You would be starving in a sea of food. Humans come equipped with a backup system for emergency access to energy just in case we find ourselves starving to death (or on a low-carbohydrate diet – but more about that later). Because the lack of insulin prevents our body from 'seeing' the carbohydrates we have just eaten, our body, convinced that we are starving, switches to Plan B – eat our own fat and muscles until somebody finds some real food. Fat and muscle mass are converted to an alternate fuel called ketones.

At this point in my reading a light went on for me. A diabetic's body thinks it's starving because it can't see the glucose in the bloodstream. Simply put, the glucose gets there because the person ate carbohydrates. If I didn't eat carbohydrates in the first place then it's likely that exactly the same effect would be produced. My body would think it was starving, switch to Plan B and start actually using up some of my (vast) supply of fat rather than storing more. This explained why low-carbohydrate diets such as Atkins work. I read further.

Born in Ohio in 1930, Robert Atkins graduated from Cornell Medical College in 1955 and commenced practice as a cardiologist in New York. In 1963, he got the kind of shock most of us run into at some point. He saw an old photo of himself from two decades earlier, when he had weighed about 15kg less. Spurred into action, he started looking into what the medical literature had to say about the latest and greatest in weight-loss techniques. He tried a couple of different diets without any real success, until he read an article in the *Journal of the American Medical Association*. The article was by Dr John Yudkin, head of the brand-new Department of Nutrition at London's Queen Elizabeth College. Dr Yudkin's study showed that a diet with unlimited protein and fat but little or no carbohydrates was much more effective than a diet that controlled calories or fat intake. Yudkin's article went on to say that when you told people not to eat carbohydrates, but to eat as much fat and protein as they liked, they actually ate up to 55 per cent fewer calories overall. All of the subjects ate less fat, some massively so. All of them lost weight. Yudkin concluded that low-carbohydrate diets worked principally because they reduced overall calorie consumption.

Dr Yudkin's study was then the most recent in a series of research projects aimed at proving or disproving the miraculous effects of the Banting diet, the first diet to suggest that people reduce carbohydrate intake. Almost 100 years to the day before Robert Atkins started looking for a solution to his middle-age spread, an English undertaker and coffin maker by the name of William Banting had solved his 'corpulence' problem by limiting his intake of carbohydrates. Born in 1797, when Banting entered his thirties he encountered a problem that was much rarer then than it is now. He started to become overweight. He was advised to increase his 'bodily exertion', which he duly did by rowing on the nearby river for two hours a day. But all this seemed to do was make him even hungrier, which meant that he ate more and became fatter. His medical friends advised him to stop exercising immediately and limit himself to moderate and light food. This he did, only to find that he was constantly hungry and broke out in boils (which sounds like a lot of the diets I tried – perhaps without the boils). Over the next 20 years he tried swimming, walking, taking the sea air, soaking himself at the spa, starvation diets and Turkish baths, but succeeded in losing just 2.5kg. By 1862, at 5 feet 5 inches (165cm), Banting weighed in at almost 100kg – hardly noteworthy by today's standards, but in 1860s England, he would have stood out as being particularly obese.

In August 1862, at the age of 65 and worried about his increasing deafness, Banting consulted Dr William Harvey, a noted ear, nose and throat specialist. When Banting appeared in his office complaining of deafness, Dr Harvey was just as interested in his story of failed diet after failed diet as he was in curing his hearing problem. Harvey also thought that the deafness may well be caused by Banting's obesity, so he suggested a diet based on the theories of Dr Claude Bernard, who thought that the liver might produce a sugar-like substance made from the fats, sugars and starches consumed as part of a 'normal' diet. Dr Harvey asked Banting to avoid bread, butter, milk, sugar, beer, pork and potatoes. This is a strange list to modern eyes, but what Dr Harvey was restricting was what doctors at the time thought were foods containing 'starch' (carbohydrates). He could eat as much meat or fruit as he wished.

Almost immediately, Banting began losing weight and generally feeling much healthier. Over the next year he lost weight at a constant rate of about half a kilo a week. A man who had failed miserably for 30 years to lose weight was suddenly able to lose 26kg in the space of a single year and cure his deafness. Banting found that, unlike all the other diets, he didn't need any willpower to stay on this one – he could eat until he was full and genuinely enjoyed his food. The only adjustment he had to make was to avoid the list of foods Dr Harvey had given him. Banting was ecstatic. He was determined that others suffering the 'oppression of corpulence' needed to know his secret, so he funded and published a book detailing his experience. He never charged for the book because he didn't want to be accused of doing it for the money.

The Banting diet was so contrary to contemporary thinking on weight loss that the medical profession immediately set against Banting and Dr Harvey. Dr Harvey was not able to provide much of a defence. He knew the diet worked but he was unable to explain why. The public didn't care why; repeated successes with the Banting diet were becoming newsworthy – or at least gossip-worthy – events, much to the frustration of the medical profession. Enter Dr Felix Neimeyer from Stuttgart. All doctors at the time 'knew' that protein was not fattening; it was only fat and starch that caused you to gain weight. It was thought that fat and starch combined with oxygen in the lungs to produce energy, with any excess becoming body fat. Neimeyer reckoned that the reason Banting's diet worked was because it restricted fat and starch. Neimeyer created a modified version that insisted on the meat being trimmed of all fat. Banting had never actually concerned himself with fat intake, but this tiny modification made the Neimeyer variation of the Banting diet instantly acceptable to the doctors.

Banting lived to the ripe old age of 81 at a normal weight and in good health. He was always very critical of the Neimeyer modification to his diet because he said it unnecessarily complicated what was quite a simple eating program. But in the end Neimeyer helped Banting's diet to gain the support of many in the medical profession and ultimately ensured that it helped many more people than those able to obtain one of the 2500 copies of his book. The Banting diet became so popular among the upper classes of Victorian England that being 'on the bant' became synonymous with dieting well into the 1920s and '30s. Those who speak Swedish will also recognise *banta* as the verb for 'diet'.

Banting's diet was copied many times before Dr Atkins read about it in the late '60s. In 1960, it was promoted as the 'Canadian Air Force Diet'; in 1964, the 'Drinking Man's Diet'; and in 1967, the 'Doctor's Quick Weight-Loss Diet'. This last diet, also known as the Stillman diet after its creator, required the dieter to eat nothing (and I mean nothing) but protein. Absolutely no fats and no carbohydrates were permitted. The Stillman diet was extraordinarily popular in its time, with the book describing the diet selling over 5.5 million copies. All of these diets had their little quirks, but they all had something in common: low or no carbohydrates. They had one other thing in common: like poor old Dr Harvey, the medical profession couldn't provide any reasonable explanation for why the diet should work, the theory of fat and starch being combined in the lungs having long since fallen by the wayside.

After reading Dr Yudkin's research, and still having difficulty fitting into his graduation pants, Atkins decided to give low-carb a try. He experienced the same persistent success enjoyed by Banting a century earlier. Unlike Stillman and a raft of others, Atkins thought he knew why the diet worked. It was all related to insulin production and the creation of a state of ketosis. Atkins published his book *Dr Atkins' Diet Revolution* in 1972, which promoted his new variation on the by then very old low-carbohydrate theme. What was unique about Atkins' book was not so much the diet itself as the considerable effort put into describing the metabolic processes that explained how the diet worked.

If Dr Atkins thought he was onto a 5.5 million bestseller, like Stillman just five years earlier, he was about to be sadly disappointed. By 1972, fat-mania, driven in large part by Dr Ancel Keys (about whom I will have much more to say later), had well and truly infected the medical establishment. Atkins was a laughing stock for suggesting you could eat as much fat as you like. The medical profession 'knew' by then that fat was the cause of most evil. All you had to do to lose weight was reduce your fat intake and show some willpower (oh, and go to the gym with Jane Fonda).

Interest in Atkins' diet smouldered in cult followings for almost two decades. In the early 1990s a new version of his book was released. This time, however, the public was ready to listen. By then, almost twice as many people needed Dr Atkins' services – and that was after having taken the low-fat advice of the medical mainstream for two decades. The Atkins diet became a worldwide phenomenon, spawning its own series of copycats (the CSIRO diet in Australia is a recent variant that isn't quite so strict). Almost two decades down the track, low-carb has almost equalled (but not yet displaced) low-fat in the food marketer's lexicon of power marketing phrases.

Since the Atkins boom in the late '90s, the medical profession has worked very hard to prove that low-carbohydrate diets are no more effective than low-fat diets. Study after study has shown that the body is perfectly capable of getting its calories from Plan B for extended periods and there is no logic to the suggestion that feeding the body protein rather than carbohydrate should produce the results claimed by the promoters of Atkins, the Zone, the South Beach Diet, the CSIRO diet or many of the other modern versions of going on the bant. The reality is, however, that, at least in the short term, they definitely work. It seems likely to me that what Dr Yudkin discussed in the article that first inspired Dr Atkins is in fact the case. When you tell people they can eat as much fat and protein as they like, just don't have carbohydrates, they actually eat fewer calories. Think about that for minute and it's not too surprising. You can't eat fruit, bread, sugar, cereal, potatoes, pasta or pastry. Bacon and eggs sounds good for breakfast but that wears very thin after even a week of having it every day – and anyway, who's got time for that palaver every morning? You can't even get it as a bacon and egg muffin on the way to work unless you plan to eat the contents and throw away the muffin. You can't have sandwiches for lunch and you can't have potatoes for dinner. Most of the things we are prepared to eat include carbohydrates to some degree. Many of these diets loosen the reins a little and let you keep eating limited carbohydrates, but if you follow those diets you are not really enacting the ketonic theory. All you are really doing is following just another calorie- or food-limiting diet.

Very recent research on the precise detail of the biochemistry of how the body turns food into energy has shown that ketonic energy production (from protein and fat) costs more in terms of calories used than 'normal' carbohydrate energy production. This means that low-carb diets should produce weight loss as long as you don't eat more of other foods to compensate for the energy drain. And Dr Yudkin's observations seemed to show that, if anything, you would eat less.

My own personal experience with low-carb diets lined up with what Dr Yudkin had found. It definitely worked, and I suspect it was because I actually ended up eating less of everything. After two days of feeling extraordinarily hungry no matter how much protein or fat I ate, my body suddenly turned off the hunger signal – as I was about to find out, the feeling of hunger is closely related to the operation of our carbohydrate regulation system. From that point on, I didn't feel particularly hungry even if I ate nothing for a whole day. My body had ample supplies of fat to keep me going for months, years or probably even decades. The trouble was that the types of food I could eat became very limited. If you rule out everything containing carbohydrates you are left with pretty much meat, dairy and salad. And believe me, after a few weeks of nothing but meat, dairy and salad, you get pretty sick of it.

In the past, I had stopped low-carb diets because I couldn't stand extended periods of trying to avoid bread, pasta and chippies. Now I had found out why it probably wasn't a good idea anyway. People on a low-carb diet became ketonic just like untreated diabetics – but hang on, they also eventually died. That seemed like a fairly extreme side effect.

Further reading revealed ketone production is not a bad thing in the short term. It is a natural response to starvation and it will keep us alive until we can find the next bunch of bananas. It's not, however, a good idea to use ketones as a long-term source of energy. As the ketones in the blood build up over time, the acidity of the blood increases significantly, since uric acid production is a by-product of the process that produces ketones. This eventually leads to widespread tissue damage (particularly highly sensitive tissues such as those involved with eyesight and the kidneys), multiple organ failure and eventually death. High blood sugar won't kill you instantly, but within a few months your muscles will begin to waste, and within a few years ketonic acidity (or ketoacidosis, if you want to get technical) will eventually lead to significant organ damage, accompanied by blindness, and then coma and ultimately death.

Hmm, definitely a good idea to leave the Atkins diet on hold. But I wasn't entirely unconvinced. It might not be necessary to eat yak steaks fed on Swiss glacial water or whatever other fandangled twist every new low-carb diet came out with, but there seemed to be good reasons why a sensible approach to low-carb eating could well produce the solid results observed by so many since Mr Banting. I parked that thought in the back of my mind and decided to find out more about metabolism.

3. HOW WE TURN FOOD INTO ENERGY

In nature, edible food is sometimes difficult to obtain. Evolution has ensured that our digestive systems are designed not to waste one calorie of the energy we put into our mouths. If glucose, and therefore energy, can be extracted, then our bodies will extract it and either use it immediately or store it for later. We can store about four hours' worth of energy as glucose in our bloodstream. This explains why we position mealtimes at equidistant times during our waking hours. So that we don't have to get up in the middle of the night to have another meal, we also make another hormone called serotonin, which is released while we are asleep. It tells our stomach we don't need to eat right now. As you might imagine, a hormone that tells us not to eat is of enormous interest to researchers in the weight-loss industry – but more on that later.

If we eat more than four hours' worth of food (because we managed to come across a particularly large dead antelope at lunchtime, for example), our bodies have a couple of energy-storage systems to deal with the extra food. I understood this a lot better when I thought of myself as being like a laptop computer. I am a top-of-the-range laptop (of course) with a nice long four-hour battery life (the equivalent of the amount of energy I can store in my bloodstream). Three times a day I plug into the mains for just long enough to charge the battery. But I also have a bag full of spare batteries. If I have access to multiple power points at my recharge time, I can charge up some of the spare batteries, just in case I'm not able to get to a mains supply in a further four hours' time. Mind you, I have to be prepared to carry around a bag of spare batteries just in case. Just like the laptop with the bag of spare batteries, we can store a further 20 hours of energy (five extra batteries) as a form of solid glucose called glycogen (often called animal starch by nutritionists or brown fat by butchers). It is stored primarily around the liver and muscles.

The liver is the second-largest organ in your body (your skin is the largest). It is the functional equivalent of a pool filter in the body, cleaning the blood supply by removing excess nutrients and poisons absorbed through the stomach and intestinal walls. One of the most important functions of the liver is to manage, recharge and discharge our short-term energy storage (our spare batteries). If insulin is in the bloodstream (usually because we have just eaten), the liver uses the insulin in a chemical reaction that sucks glucose out of the bloodstream and converts it to long chains of glucose molecules, which are stored as glycogen. Just in case you are keeping a list of all these Greek and Latin words, the medical term for this process is glycogenesis, but I wouldn't bother remembering that unless you plan to become an endocrinologist (or have easily impressed acquaintances). Stored glucose in the form of glycogen helps us to smooth out our energy requirements. Without it, we would have to eat every four hours or run the very real risk of running out of the

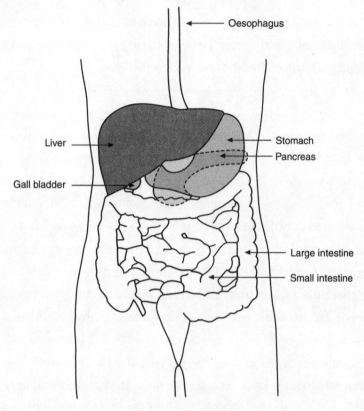

Oesophagus

Liver

Gall bladder

Stomach

Pancreas

Large intestine

Small intestine

Figure 3.1: The liver is the dark grey-coloured organ in this picture.

glucose fuel required to keep our brain and internal organs functioning. Glycogen stores give us the fast-burn capacity to keep going for up to 24 hours without having to eat at all.

Insulin is such an important protein that it is common to all animals. It works in exactly the same way in worms and fish as it does in mammals. There is only a three-amino-acid difference (out of 51) between cow insulin and human insulin. Pig insulin is an even better match, with only a one-amino-acid differential. Today, sufferers of diabetes don't inject pig, cow and fish insulin; they inject manufactured human insulin. In 1982, Eli Lilly introduced a genetically

engineered copy of human insulin, which has since spawned many
similar preparations, and it is now illegal to use anything other than
synthetic human insulin in many countries.

Glycogen is not the only energy-storage system we have. We
also have the ability to store excess energy as fat (and don't we all
know about that). Once again, insulin is the trigger for this mechanism. Just as normal cells need insulin to convert glucose to energy,
fat cells need insulin to convert glucose to fat. So, as well as helping
cells that need energy to access the glucose, and converting glucose
to glycogen, the third way that insulin helps us reduce the circulating glucose load is to help the fat cells pack away any excess glucose
as body fat. Fat is almost twice as dense as carbohydrate or protein;
a kilogram of body fat stores almost double the energy that a kilo
of muscle or glycogen does. If you stored all excess energy as glycogen rather than fat, it would take up almost twice as much space
and weigh almost twice as much. (I'll bet that's the first time you've
thought of body fat as being a good thing.) Getting back to my laptop analogy, body fat is like a super-long-life battery that takes twice
as long to charge but also lasts twice as long (and only weighs the
same as the other batteries).

The good news from a survival perspective is that, unlike circulating blood sugar or glycogen, you can store virtually unlimited
amounts of body fat (well, in theory). It also means that your body
is designed to take every opportunity to store body fat, because you
never know when you'll bring down your next antelope.

At about this point in my reading another light went on in my
head. So that was why I kept getting fatter – I was designed to eat all
available food and store it as body fat. Maybe there were diets that
reduced the amount of insulin released after a meal, which would

mean that less fat was stored? I started looking and it wasn't long before I stumbled onto GI diets. GI stands for glycaemic index and, simply put, it is a measure of the degree to which any given food produces a spike in blood sugar (and therefore insulin). It's kind of like the different types of fuel you can feed a fire. If you put pine planks on the fire, they will burn very hot and very quickly but they will be used up in minutes. If, however, you put hardwood sleepers on, they will burn slowly for hours. Low-GI foods are hardwood sleepers to our body and high-GI foods are pine planks. GI diets effectively treat all of us like we are suffering from diabetes – the theory is that if you aim to keep blood-glucose levels and therefore insulin levels low and constant, your appetite will be largely suppressed and large quantities of insulin will not be released and used to create body fat.

It sounded logical to me, so I immediately started reading about the glycaemic index and looking for low-GI foods.

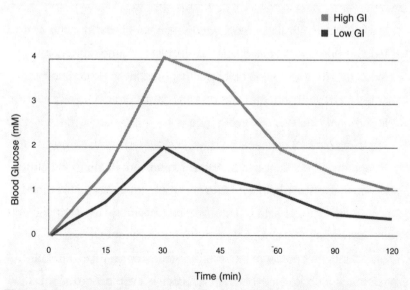

Figure 3.2: A comparison of the effect that the GI of a food will have on blood-glucose levels over time. High-GI foods cause a much higher spike than low-GI foods.

In 1981 in the *American Journal of Clinical Nutrition*, Dr David Jenkins, a professor of Nutritional Science at the University of Toronto, was the first to publish a theory about the glycaemic index and its effect on diet. Dr Jenkins developed the index to help doctors determine what foods were best for diabetics. He found that there was no simple rule such as 'don't eat potatoes' or 'do eat meat'; rather, all foods produced different blood-sugar responses based on the combination of carbohydrates, fats and proteins, as well as how much indigestible fibre was present. It was, however, left to an Australian to develop a comprehensive tabulation of the glycaemic index of almost 600 foods. Dr Jennie Brand-Miller, an associate professor and head of the teaching and research staff of the Human Nutrition Unit of the Department of Biochemistry at the University of Sydney, became the most vocal champion of using GI ratings to assess foods when she published her book *The GI Factor* in 1996.

Unlike fat, protein and carbohydrate measures, the GI value of a food is relatively difficult to calibrate. It relies on feeding volunteers foods and measuring their blood-sugar responses. This is complicated by the fact that the response will differ from day to day even in the same person. To avoid inconsistency, the best measures are taken over 10 consecutive days and averaged over a group of volunteers. The volunteers are given an amount of the food being tested that will deliver exactly 50g of carbohydrate. So, for example, if we were testing pasta (25 per cent carbohydrate) we would give the volunteers 200g of pasta to eat). Scientists then compare the blood-sugar response of the volunteer to the pasta with a standard reference food for that volunteer (glucose is the most common).

Previously doctors thought that complex carbohydrates like potatoes and rice were absorbed slowly. GI measurements prove this is not so. Rice has a glycaemic index of 94 (where pure glucose is 100), which means that it is very high and will produce an immediate spike in blood sugar. Pasta has a low glycaemic index because it is prepared from cracked wheat, not from wheat flour. The method of preparation makes a difference to the particle size and therefore to the speed at which we can absorb it. To make matters worse, cooking the food will sometimes change the glycaemic index. Cooked pasta has a higher index than raw pasta, and you can lower the index of any food by adding fat or fibre to it, since both add weight to the food and lower the percentage of the food that is carbohydrate. Remember, the GI only measures the body's response to carbohydrates.

At first this diet looked like a great idea to me; the problem was that it was very hard to guess what the GI of any food was going to be, and I wasn't prepared to walk around a supermarket with Dr Brand-Miller's 600-item list in my hands. Fortunately, I was not on my own in wanting GI information, and some food manufacturers were starting to label their foods with GI values. There was a range of low-GI breads, and even chocolate drinks and spreads had low-GI labels . . . Hang on a sec! What kind of diet was this that encouraged you to drink a chocolate drink that is half sugar and eat a chocolate spread that is half fat and a third sugar?

I quickly realised that food manufacturers had figured out that they could label their food low GI because the fat content lowered the GI rating dramatically. I very much doubted that it was Dr Brand-Miller's intent to develop a plan to allow you to eat significant quantities of fat and sugar and call it a diet. GI would obviously be important to a diabetic needing to keep blood-sugar readings in check, but I struggled with the notion that our predecessors were controlling their blood sugar through some intuitive sense of the GI of the foods they encountered on the plains and in the jungles. We must be capable (at least when healthy) of dealing with blood-sugar spikes. I couldn't believe that the only reason we were suddenly all getting fatter was that we were suddenly consuming more potatoes and less pasta (and chocolate spread). It just didn't stack up logically. Clearly I needed to find out more about how our bodies deal with carbohydrates – and stop eating chocolate spread and calling it a diet.

It turns out that insulin is the Swiss army knife of hormones. It doesn't just help cells to make energy and help the liver and fat cells to store energy. It also has some appetite control properties – it stops us eating when we have taken on sufficient energy. Once insulin is introduced into our bloodstream it interacts with special receptor cells in a part of our brain called the hypothalamus.

The hypothalamus is a critical and very complex central control unit for the human body. Some of the major things it controls are our growth, our body temperature, when we sleep, our thirst and, most importantly for this discussion, our hunger.

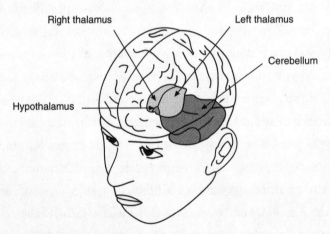

Figure 3.3: The almond-sized hypothalamus is the control centre for most of the body's automatic functions

The hypothalamus is continuously sampling our circulating blood. For example, when it detects foreign cells like bacteria or viruses, it turns up our body temperature in an effort to kill them. And when it detects insulin in the blood it tells our brain we have had enough to eat. Another part of the hypothalamus then tells the brain to reduce food intake. If the part of the hypothalamus controlling food intake is surgically removed in laboratory animals, the animal stops eating altogether. (While this is probably an effective dietary control it's a little irreversible, so put down that scalpel.) Cut out the part that detects insulin and the animal becomes obese. As much as we like to think we are in control of what and when we eat, it seems to be an unconscious choice controlled by a lump of nerve cells that wouldn't cover a postage stamp.

This insulin-induced fullness signal only works for as long as there is excess insulin circulating in the blood, so it is relatively short term. It is enough to make us push back from the table with the feeling of a full and satisfied tummy. We can consciously fight the fullness signal and eat on regardless (and if this was the only meal we had had for a few days, we probably would). In the normal course, however, it seems we are designed to stop when we have had enough, so there goes my 'perpetual eating leads to fatness' theory. Fat and glycogen storage are really just smoothing and backup systems for storage of occasional excess energy. It seems insulin's interaction with our hypothalamus would normally ensure we never ate too much more than we needed.

To maintain that full feeling for longer than an hour or so after eating, insulin also triggers the release of the hormone leptin, another long-term appetite suppressant. Leptin is a relative newcomer to our understanding of human appetite. It was first discovered just 13 years ago by Dr Jeffrey Friedman at Rockefeller University, a private institution based in New York City dedicated to biomedical research.

Dr Friedman found that obese mice were missing a gene, which he christened the ob (obese) gene. Not having the ob gene meant the mice could not produce a hormone that Friedman named leptin (from the Greek *leptos*, meaning thin). When the obese mice were continuously injected with leptin, they quickly reverted to normal body size. As you can imagine, the announcement of an injectable substance that made obese mice thin again made just a few headlines in 1995. Unfortunately, subsequent human trials revealed that it only really worked as a cure for obesity if you were one of the very, very, very small group of humans with the same genetic mutation as those mice (meaning you didn't have an ob gene). By 1998, the researchers were pretty much satisfied that injecting the rest of us with leptin was unlikely to cure obesity.

Leptin is produced by fat cells in response to the presence of circulating insulin. The more insulin in your bloodstream, the more leptin will be produced. Because insulin is swiftly eliminated from the bloodstream by the various digestive processes, the body requires a longer-term means of appetite control. Leptin performs that longer-term function. The insulin gets used up doing other jobs, like converting glucose to fat and energy, but the leptin stays around, continuing to tell the hypothalamus that we are still full. If it weren't for leptin, the feeling of fullness created by insulin after a meal would not last. We would begin to feel hungry again as soon as circulating insulin was used up (an hour or so after a meal).

Since leptin is produced by fat cells, the more fat you have, the more leptin you will generally have in your bloodstream. In this way, leptin acts like a fat meter for the hypothalamus. Lots of fat translates to lots of leptin, which in turn results in suppressed appetite for longer periods. Theoretically, if you are carrying a little extra, leptin should moderate your food intake over the longer term and you should gradually use up your fat stores. It's a very elegant design; the only trouble is that something about it is clearly not working because we are all getting fatter.

A raft of recent studies have clearly shown that high levels of fatty acids in the arteries block the action of leptin in much the same way that they inhibit insulin. Insulin resistance means that your immediate appetite control is impaired and will eventually lead to type II diabetes (see chapters 8 and 9). Leptin resistance means that your body loses the ability to tell when it has had enough to eat over the medium to long term. If you don't know you are full, you just keep eating until suddenly you realise your wedding suit doesn't fit any more.

4. USING STORED ENERGY

About four hours after we eat (unless we are asleep and therefore using less energy) glucose concentrations in our blood will begin to fall below a lower threshold. Once again, the change in glucose concentration is detected by our pancreas. But this time, instead of releasing insulin into the blood, it releases a hormone called glucagon.

In 1923, shortly after insulin was discovered, Professor John Murlin at the University of Rochester, New York, noticed that when the pancreatic extracts were injected into diabetic patients, there was a brief, but noticeable, spike in glucose levels just before the insulin acted to reduce them. He speculated that there might be another hormone in the pancreatic extracts that had the opposite effect to insulin. He (quite confusingly) called this hormone glucagon, which is not to be mixed up with glycogen, the solid form of glucose stored around the liver. Glucagon was proved to be a hormone in 1959 and its role in diabetes was confirmed in the '60s and '70s. By 1985, its role in the digestive system was well understood.

Glucagon is best thought of as anti-insulin because its effects are almost exactly the opposite of those of insulin. Its purpose is to get glucose concentrations back up to normal levels. If your blood-glucose levels fall the results can be disastrous and, unlike with high blood glucose, immediate. Glucose is your fuel. If you run out, you stop. The end. It's that simple. Too little glucose, called hypoglycaemia (*hypo* – too little; *glyc* – sugar; *aemia* – in the blood), results in very immediate problems for your brain. Remember, the only fuel your brain can use is pure glucose. Without it, the brain begins to shut down. At first mental efficiency decreases, then shakiness and sudden depression occur (hypoglycaemic diabetics can sometimes be mistaken for drunks when they reach this point), followed quickly by coma and then death. Type 1 diabetics can no more manufacture glucagon than they can insulin. If they inject too much insulin, they run the real risk of suffering hypoglycaemic shock. Blood sugar can be quickly raised simply by eating anything containing glucose, which is why this type of diabetic likes to have ready access to sweets in case they start to feel dizzy.

For the rest of us, glucagon is a pretty important safety mechanism. To restore our blood-glucose levels to a normal range, it does a number of things. Firstly, it instructs our liver to access our short-term energy store by telling it to convert glycogen stores back into circulating glucose. This is the chemical equivalent of changing batteries on my laptop. Glucagon tells the liver to go into reverse, stop storing glucose and instead start using it. That solves the emergency need for glucose and should keep us alive long enough to find something new to eat. Remember that, if we are fully charged, we have a good 20 to 24 hours of emergency power stored around our liver as glycogen. But it doesn't stop there: glucagon also tells the liver to convert amino acids (the component parts of proteins) into glucose, and tells our fat cells to release energy. The fat cells release the fatty acids they stored in better times and the presence of glucagon allows them to be separated from their glycerol backbone. The glycerol is then converted to glucose for use as fuel.

But if that were all the hormone did, we would be blissfully unaware because our leptin levels would still be telling our brain that we were full. If something weren't done to tell us to look for food, we'd still die, we'd just last a bit longer while we ran down our spare batteries. To stop this from happening, glucagon also stimulates the production of a hormone in the stomach called ghrelin.

With the discovery of leptin, the hunt was on for the appetite-stimulating hormone that was leptin's counterpart. Researchers knew that if the hormone could be identified, it might be possible to suppress its effects in some way. A multi-billion-dollar market beckoned for a drug that could suppress appetite and in the mid-1990s there were plenty of people looking. A team at Merck Pharmaceuticals knew that such a hormone must exist, because in 1994 they had identified the receptors for it in the hypothalamus. Research teams were furiously testing tissue samples from organs all over the body to attempt to isolate the hormone that instructed the hypothalamus to make us hungry. Most teams were searching the hypothalamus itself, but in 1999, Masayasu Kojima and Kenji Kangawa at Japan's National Cardiovascular Centre just pipped the Merck team at the post and found ghrelin.

The hormone they discovered gets its strange name because it interacts with the growth hormone receptor (GHR) in the hypothalamus. Kojima and Kangawa found it in massive quantities in the stomach lining (in retrospect, not an entirely strange place to look for something that makes the tummy rumble at dinnertime). Ghrelin is produced by the stomach lining in response to the presence of glucagon in the bloodstream, blocking the action of insulin (and leptin) in the hypothalamus. Circulating leptin levels stay reasonably constant most of the time, so our default appetite position is that we are full (or at least not hungry). Ghrelin counteracts the effect of leptin on the hypothalamus, effectively neutralising leptin for a while so we can feel hungry. The release of ghrelin is like throwing a 'hungry' switch in our brain. Ghrelin also stimulates our stomachs to contract, giving us that empty gurgling feeling that tells us it's time to eat.

Not surprisingly, there has been a lot of research into a 'vaccine' for ghrelin. Between 1999 and 2002, there were no fewer than 130 published research articles on ghrelin (40 of which were co-authored by Kangawa). The theory is that if you could block ghrelin's interaction with the hypothalamus, you'd never feel hungry and, therefore, you wouldn't eat and wouldn't get fat. Dr Kim Janda from the Scripps Research Institute in La Jolla, California, published results in 2007 of successful animal testing of a vaccine that trains the immune system to identify and destroy ghrelin. In other words, treat the hormone that makes us hungry like a bacterial infection and train the body to kill it. Now, that sounds good in theory, but the one thing I have noticed about hormones in all my reading is that they often do much more than one thing. Remember leptin? Injecting it was supposed to stop you getting hungry too. It turns out it doesn't work quite that way, because it seems that almost none of us has a defective ob gene. Nevertheless, if you feel like turning your body into a lab experiment, you won't have to wait long. Human trials of a ghrelin vaccine will probably have commenced by the time you are reading this.

In a healthy body, insulin and glucagon act in opposing fashion to keep our blood-glucose levels (our fuel supply) at constant levels. Each of these important hormones will trigger either the storage (insulin) or use (glucagon) of the body's short- and long-term energy stores, as well as act on the appetite centre in the brain to tell us whether to start or stop eating. The insulin/glucagon feedback loop is designed to keep us on an even keel, consuming just enough energy to keep our body running at the level of activity we choose to pursue. In common with all other animals, we are designed to maintain a normal healthy weight in all but exceptional circumstances.

Remember, in a normal diet our energy needs are supplied by carbohydrate, protein (predominantly from meat) and fat. Your body needs fats to function properly. Dietary fat is made up of a variety of fatty acids bonded to a backbone of glycerol. When we eat fat, it is absorbed by our upper intestine and transported into our bloodstream as triacylglycerols (three fatty acids tied together by glycerol, a sugar alcohol of glucose), sometimes called TCGs, lipids or fatty acids. The fatty acids are used in the production of cell membranes (our brain is almost all fat) and are critical for the production of several hormones, which help regulate blood pressure, heart rate, blood-vessel constriction and blood clotting. Fatty acids are also important for the transportation of fat-soluble vitamins (vitamins A, D, E and K) around our body. Unused circulating fatty acids are eventually converted back into stored body fat.

When we eat fat or protein, our upper intestine releases a hormone called cholecystokinin (which thankfully gets abbreviated to CCK), from the Greek *chole* – bile; *cysto* – sac; and *kinin* – move; technically, 'move the bile sac'. CCK was originally discovered in 1928 and was known to induce contractions in the gall bladder, the small organ between the liver and the pancreas (see page 27, Figure 3.1). It's a sac that contains a reserve of about 50ml of bile.

Bile is used to emulsify any fat that enters our stomach. Researchers have known since 1928 that CCK triggers the release of digestive enzymes from the pancreas and bile from the gall bladder. Only in the last decade has it become clear that in much the same way as leptin does, CCK also tells the hypothalamus to suppress hunger and make us feel full.

We have a well-developed system for accurately detecting when we have had exactly as much food as we need. Carbohydrates and proteins are regulated using the insulin/glucagon control of blood glucose, and fats are regulated by the similar use of CCK. I was once told that modern passenger aircraft constantly cycle fuel between their wing and fuselage tanks to ensure that the plane is always perfectly balanced as the fuel is used up. The fuel-management system at work in your body makes that system look about as modern as Fred Flintstone's car. Right now, your body is delicately adjusting hormone levels to cycle multiple energy stores up or down based on the energy you need, when you last ate, what you ate and when you last slept (among other things). All of that is happening without you having to think about it at all (thank goodness – I'm flat out balancing a cheque book, let alone doing all that). It is a truly elegant design, but it is one that is wholly dependent on the assumption that the environment that 'designed' it is still the same as when it was put together.

5. FAT MAKES YOU FAT . . .
OR DOES IT?

We are thin by design. If we are eating the diet our digestive system is designed to use, one dominated by foods that are compounds of glucose or can be converted to glucose, the insulin/glucagon (for carbohydrates and proteins) and CCK (for fats) feedback loops will keep us thin. We will eat only when we are hungry and we will store minimal additional body fat. We come equipped with a fully functioning calorie detector, the hypothalamus. It has no need for calorie tables or calculators to determine how much food we need or how much fat we have stored on the body. It has been designed by millions of years of evolution to accurately and elegantly count and control our energy intake so that we maintain optimal body weight.

So, if we are so perfectly designed, how do we get fat? If you read all the reports of the experiments each of these researchers did in discovering the effects of each of the hormones they uncovered, it becomes very clear that obesity and anorexia were very simply induced (or cured) in the animals they were studying. All they had to do was chop this bit off or inject a bit more of that. The will-power of the animal seemed to have very little to do with whether it decided to eat or not. There was no need to send them off to the mouse gym or enrol them in *The Biggest Loser*. Their appetite and therefore their weight was all very simply controlled by changing the hormone mix. Assuming humans are running to the same blue-print, and nothing in the research suggests we aren't, there must be something else besides lack of willpower at play in making us fat.

For decades, governments and doctors alike have been telling us that the 'something' that is making us fat is quite obviously fat. When doctors first started looking for explanations for why we were suddenly getting fat, the obvious candidate for an increase in body fat was increasing consumption of foods containing fat. After all, that sounds intuitively logical, and fat consumption was increasing roughly in line with the increase in human body fat production. In 1909 the average American was consuming just over 14kg of fat every year. By 2001 this had almost tripled after a significant spike in the '90s.

The 'fat makes you fat' message was first promoted by Dr Ancel Keys. In 1939, Keys joined the Mayo Foundation, run by the University of Minnesota in Rochester, Minnesota, where he created a new division of biochemical research on human beings, Human Physiology and Biochemistry. The following year he was invited to organise what was to become the Laboratory of Physiological Hygiene at the university's main campus in Minneapolis. By this time, World War II was engulfing Europe and America's involvement was becoming more certain by the day. The US Department of Defense was one of the biggest-paying customers of Keys' new lab, and one of his first contracts was to run subsistence tests for the Department. His task was to determine the least amount of food required to keep a

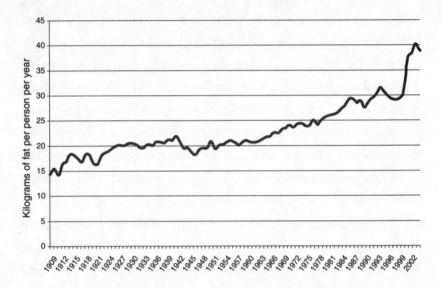

Figure 5.1: This graph is based on data from the USDA (US Department of Agriculture). An obvious cause of the obesity epidemic is fat consumption, said the researchers, and graphs like this show we clearly are eating more fat – but is it really the cause?

combat soldier alive and in fighting condition. By 1941, Keys was serving as special assistant to the Secretary of War; his primary role was to develop rations for combat troops. Keys and his team had scoured the local supermarket to create what was essentially a lunch box full of high-calorie, long-life foods. The infamous K-rations ('K' for Keys) became – and remain, albeit heavily modified – a staple of the US military.

As the end of the war approached, Keys began to realise that starvation was going to be a significant problem in Europe when the fighting stopped. He obtained funding and resources for the Minnesota Starvation Experiment, in which he and his team fed volunteers half the normal number of calories for adult males, while ensuring that they kept up a normal exercise regime. The idea was to put the volunteers on a diet that simulated what life was like in the war-torn remains of Europe. On average, each man lost 25 per cent of his body weight, 10 per cent of muscle strength and 50 per cent of endurance over the five months of the study.

The starvation studies gave Keys access to significant population and food data coming out of post-war Europe. Looking at this data, Keys noticed that as food supplies reached starvation levels, the death rate from coronary heart disease dropped significantly. Keys couldn't explain that counterintuitive observation. Surely more people should be dying of heart attacks as they starved, not fewer? Keys developed a theory to explain the data. He thought that a full-calorie diet contained more fat and therefore more cholesterol than a starvation diet. If there is too much cholesterol in the blood, it can accumulate and cause arterial blockages (atherosclerosis), which can lead to heart attack or stroke. The elimination of fat in the starvation diet would therefore mean that patients would have less heart disease. Keys' theory that there was a correlation between dietary fat and heart disease was just a theory, and it was based on only a few observations, so, by then a very influential researcher, he obtained funding to launch a long-range study aimed at determining the factors involved in 'degeneration of the heart'. He recruited 286 Minnesota businessmen and set up a metabolic research unit at a local hospital.

By the time Keys started his study in 1953, it was well known that the build-up of cholesterol (Greek for solid bile) was a major cause of some types of heart disease. Cholesterol, a fatty substance manufactured by our liver, provides material for the repair of cell walls and the manufacture of some hormones. It is critical to normal brain and nerve function and is used as a transport mechanism to carry fatty acids in the bloodstream. Over time, cholesterol deposits build up on artery walls. When the cholesterol build-up entirely blocks an artery supplying blood to the heart wall, a heart attack can occur.

Dr Keys' study of the Minnesota businessmen was a precursor to his more elaborate Seven Countries Study, which launched in 1958 and ran for the following decade. The now famous study examined data on the diets of a selection of different countries and seemed to show that the higher the level of fat in a nation's diet, the greater its rate of heart disease. Keys explained the results by suggesting that a diet rich in saturated fat, found in animal products such as meat, eggs and dairy products, produces higher levels of cholesterol in the blood. This, in turn, increases the risk of the artery-furring process that gives rise to heart disease. The obvious outward symptom of all this fat consumption is weight gain.

From the mid-1950s, Keys actively promoted his theory to an increasingly health-conscious public. With his wife, Margaret, Keys popularised the 'Mediterranean diet' with a series of bestselling books. The diet is based on mimicking the food intake of Mediterranean and Asian cultures that scored well on the Seven Countries Study. Dr Keys must have been doing something right because he lived to the ripe old age of 101, passing on peacefully in his sleep at the end of 2004. Keys is probably almost single-handedly responsible for the five decades of product marketing directed towards low-fat foods that followed the publication of his famous study.

The case against saturated fat and cholesterol was, however, probably not as open-and-shut as Keys and his followers would have us believe. When Dr Keys published his study, he focused on just seven countries. But at that time, data from 22 countries existed, which may suggest Keys was perhaps a little selective about the evidence he decided to include. In the study, Keys produced a graph with the amount of fat in the food of the seven countries plotted on one axis and the average blood-cholesterol levels for those countries plotted on the other axis. In Dr Keys' graph, the data points (fat in the diet versus cholesterol) fell on a straight line. Mathematically this meant that fat consumption and cholesterol were beautifully correlated for those seven countries. Using that single graph, Keys drew the conclusion that dietary fat consumption caused high blood cholesterol. That conclusion became an easy-to-digest (pardon the pun) message that half a century of low-cholesterol marketing has ingrained as modern health fact beyond dispute. Fat makes you fat. If data points from the fifteen countries that Dr Keys failed to include are added to his graph, the correlation appears far less convincing and the conclusion that there is any relationship between dietary fat consumption and cholesterol or obesity correspondingly more difficult to maintain.

Even within the data presented by Keys there were significant problems. For instance, despite similar fat intakes, heart disease deaths in Finland were found to be seven times higher than in Mexico. The Mediterranean island of Crete was an even more astounding aberration. With almost 40 per cent of the calorie intake of Cretan participants coming from fat, they experienced the lowest death rates of all countries studied. Professor Keys explained these aberrations by theorising that, unlike the saturated animal fat that was in American and Finnish diets, the majority of the fat in the Cretan diet came from olive oil and fish, which are rich in unsaturated fats. Keys concluded that, although saturated fat can be harmful to your health, unsaturated fats can have positive health benefits. Subsequent studies have also found enormous variance in heart disease rates within countries, despite consistent blood-cholesterol levels.

Keys' message to avoid saturated fat and you would stop being fat certainly had a simple logic. Brilliant marketing by Keys and those that followed on the 'eat less fat' bandwagon ensured that for the last three decades of the last century we were all encouraged to purchase fat-free or fat-reduced foods at every turn. Detailed studies of food consumption habits conducted by the US Department of Agriculture from 1971 to 2000 have confirmed that Keys' and his followers' message got through. During those three decades, the percentage of the food energy in the average American's diet that came from fat actually decreased (from 36.5 per cent to 32.8 per cent). The strange thing was that not only did the substantial decrease in fat consumption not result in a reduction in the average waistline, but it was expanding faster than it ever had – in fact, it had doubled. We had obeyed Dr Keys' command to eat less fat and it seemed to be making us fatter, not thinner.

I was less than convinced. If I were inclined to be mischievous with statistics, I could easily justify a message that not eating fat made you twice as fat. What I was about to discover was not so much that fat was good for me, but that, left to its own devices, my body could deal with fat in my diet. Eating fat put fatty acids in my arteries, that was for certain. But my body could tell when I had had enough fat and stop me eating more. I was about to discover that my body had no such control over fructose, and yet it just as effectively pumped fatty acids into my arteries. Even worse than that, because fructose was invisible to my appetite control, it allowed me to eat just as much fat as I normally would, and then eat as much fructose (which became fat) as I could shove into my mouth. No wonder I was getting fatter no matter how much low-fat food I purchased.

As long ago as 1977, Dr George Mann described the diet/heart idea (eating fat gives you heart disease) as the 'greatest scam in the history of medicine'. Dr Mann, a professor of Medicine and Bio-chemistry at Vanderbilt University in Tennessee, concluded after studying the Maasai people of Kenya during the early '60s that diet could not possibly influence cholesterol levels. Not unlike most of my children, the Maasai believe that vegetables are food for cows, not humans (they are cattle farmers). They each subsist on 2L of full-cream cow's milk per day and when they celebrate they do so with an orgy of meat and blood consumption, with each person eating more than 1kg of meat in a sitting. Yet Maasai tribes have the lowest cholesterol readings ever measured, on average half that of an adult American.

I knew from personal experience that going fat free made almost no visible difference to my waistline. Perhaps I was less of a heart attack waiting to happen, but based on Dr Mann's work, I doubt it. I was still fat; it was just that food was less pleasant to eat. The 'fat gives you heart disease' theory and the natural corollary (which Keys claimed was obvious), the 'fat makes you fat' theory, didn't gel with what I had discovered about our digestive system either. According to everything I had read, eating fat should have kicked in the CCK feedback loop, which would tell my hypothalamus I was full and stop me eating more than I needed. I shouldn't be able to get any fatter eating fat than I would eating carbohydrates. Sure, fat might be worse for cholesterol (I wasn't convinced about that either), but I couldn't see how it could be responsible for obesity.

Dr Cleave had said sugar was clogging up our pancreas (perhaps not exactly his words) and that the cure was more bran. I hadn't seen anything in all my reading to this point to justify a theory that sugar was affecting the pancreas (or that bran was likely to help in any way even if it was). Sugar was a food like any other and all the normal mechanisms should apply, shouldn't they? But Dr Cleave's graphs seemed to show a strong relationship between rapidly rising sugar consumption and obesity-related diseases.

As we know, unlike most carbohydrates like grains, breads and pasta, which are almost entirely glucose based, sugar is only half glucose. The other half is fructose. I theorised that perhaps the answer lay in the degree to which we were adapted to dealing with large quantities of fructose in our diet. It was time to see what the medical establishment knew about the consumption of fructose and whether it might have an effect on our weight. It was lucky I had been boning up on Greek and Latin medical terms, because if I was expecting to find anything written in plain English I was about to be very disappointed.

It immediately became apparent that I wasn't the only person questioning the evidence and the conclusions being drawn from Dr Keys' work. His detractors weren't famous Americans with a diet book to sell, so it took a little more digging to find their work. At around the same time that Surgeon-Captain Cleave and Dr Keys were working on their solutions to the obesity problem, Professor John Yudkin was taking a different tack.

Born in the East End of London in 1910, John Yudkin studied Physiology and Biochemistry at Cambridge and, while studying for his PhD, he developed an interest in nutrition. He later became a doctor, serving in the Army Medical Corps in West Africa during World War II. After the war, Yudkin was appointed Professor of Physiology at the University of London's Queen Elizabeth College (QEC), eventually establishing the first university department in the UK that offered undergraduate-level nutrition degrees. Yudkin became the School's Professor of Nutrition, a job he retained until he retired in 1971.

During the 1950s Professor Yudkin became increasingly disturbed by the obvious inconsistencies in the evidence emerging from Dr Keys' research linking animal fats to heart disease and obesity. So he began searching for another dietary factor. Because he was an expert in carbohydrate metabolism, he initially focused (like Dr Cleave) on sugar consumption because, like fat, its use was rapidly increasing. In laboratory and human tests, he found that eating table sugar increased the amount of LDL cholesterol (the 'bad' cholesterol) in the blood. But not only that, he found that all circulating fats (TCGs) generally increased. There is a growing body of evidence linking TCGs to the clogging of arteries, which may increase the risk of a heart attack or stroke. In fact, some researchers now think that TCG levels in the blood may actually be more important than cholesterol levels in establishing heart disease risk.

Professor Yudkin also noted increased uric acid levels. Remember, because of a lack of insulin in a diabetes patient, the body thinks it's starving and starts eating its own protein and fat to produce ketones, which are used for energy. The Atkins diet (or any other high-protein diet) produces the same effect by starving the body of carbohydrates, forcing it to switch to protein and fat metabolism as its primary source of energy. Uric acid is the by-product of that process. Prolonged excess uric acid production eventually leads to the high blood acidity that does so much damage to the eyes, kidneys and other fragile organs in diabetics. Doctors knew that high uric acid levels were associated with a type of arthritis called gout, renal (kidney) failure, gallstones and an increased risk of heart disease. They also knew that eating too much meat, particularly internal organs like the offal granddad used to eat, could cause uric acid levels to be higher than normal. Dr Yudkin's discovery that eating sugar could also cause high uric acid levels came as a bit of a shock.

Another unexpected increase detected by Dr Yudkin was in the hormone cortisol. Cortisol is produced by the adrenal gland (the maker of adrenaline), and is often called the stress hormone because it's released by the gland in response to stress. Cortisol gets everything working harder and faster during times of stress (which was probably particularly handy when being chased by a woolly mammoth or sabre-toothed tiger). It temporarily increases blood pressure (for faster thinking) and blood sugar (for extra energy), and suppresses the body's immune response, so energy is focused on the more immediate concern of staying alive, rather than the endless hunt for nasty infections.

Cortisol release is cyclical. Your body gives you a kick-start in the morning by squirting just a little more than normal into the blood and it tones it down when you are trying to sleep. Pretty much any time you are about to have a stressful experience (fear, pain, a meeting with your publisher, that kind of thing), cortisol levels increase. And also, Dr Yudkin somewhat surprisingly discovered, when you eat sugar. That might go a long way to explaining the 'sugar high' that every parent of young children will tell you is very real.

The other surprising change in subjects fed large amounts of sugar was that their blood became stickier; in other words, it clotted more easily. This is worth remembering, especially in the context of the fact that most cases of heart disease over the past hundred years are of a form that is new, namely heart attack or myocardial infarction – a massive blood clot leading to obstruction of a coronary artery and consequent death of the heart muscle.

Professor Yudkin's initial findings were published in 1957, the year before Dr Keys launched his famous Seven Countries Study. Yudkin and his team followed up that research during the '60s with investigations of larger populations that showed that the rise in the incidence of heart disease consistently coincided with the rise in the consumption of sugar, but could not be consistently associated with the consumption of fat, whether it was saturated or unsaturated.

As dramatic as those findings were, the real surprise came when Dr Yudkin substituted fructose for sugar in his experiments. Remember that table sugar (or sucrose) is a combination of two simpler sugars, glucose and fructose. Yudkin knew that the human body broke sugar into these constituent parts as part of the digestive process and wanted to determine whether either part had more influence on his findings. 'The effects of eating sucrose in the quantities we eat are magnified with fructose. Fructose is the dangerous part,' he said.

Dr Yudkin published a popular explanation of his concerns about sugar in 1972. His book *Sweet and Deadly* came in for sustained attack from Dr Keys, principally because it suggested that it was sugar and not fat that was the cause of heart disease. The retiring British academic was no match for the well-publicised American, and Dr Keys' theories won the day in the popular (and scientific) conscience.

Meanwhile, the US Department of Agriculture was doing some interesting things with rats. The USDA has a long and proud history in human nutrition research. In 1953, the tide of interest in human nutrition that was floating Dr Keys' boat had also inspired the USDA to establish the Agricultural Research Service, with a mission to find solutions to agricultural problems that affect everyday Americans. A key facility for the service is the Beltsville Human Nutrition Research Center in Maryland (Beltsville for short).

Dr Yudkin's warning bells on sugar (and in particular, fructose) had been muffled by the intervention of the Keys media machine, but Dr Sheldon Reiser, the lead researcher on carbohydrate metabolism at Beltsville, had been reading Yudkin's work. He decided to start feeding some hapless rats fructose-rich diets. From 1975 until his retirement in 1990, Dr Reiser published study after study that concluded without a shadow of a doubt that it was the fructose half of sugar that was doing all manner of damage in his furry subjects. On the high-fructose diet, the rats developed severe problems with vital organs. Liver, heart and testes exhibited extreme swelling, while the pancreas atrophied, invariably leading to the death of the rats. Interestingly, the damage was much greater in male rats than in females. Dr Yudkin had discovered a similar trend among the rabbits used in his experiments, and had theorised that perhaps female reproductive hormones in some way reduced the negative impacts of the sugar. He went on to verify this in limited human trials, which showed that post-menopausal women were at just as high a risk as men, but pre-menopausal women had much lower risks associated with the intake of sugar.

Emboldened by almost a decade of dead rats, and drawing some criticism about the applicability of rat studies to human consumption patterns (nobody in the US had paid much attention to Yudkin's work), Dr Reiser decided to conduct a limited human version of his experiments in 1984. The study's official goal was to investigate the effect of fructose consumption on the health of 24 men aged 21 to 57, consuming a diet marginally low in copper. Health surveys conducted by the USDA during the '70s had revealed that the average American had far too little copper in their diet, and experiments with rats had repeatedly shown that copper deficiency magnified the ill-effects of fructose, particularly in male rats. The diets used in the study were designed to represent typical American diets in both composition and size. The men were divided into two groups of 12. One group was fed a diet where 20 per cent of the calories came from fructose and the others were fed the same diet except the fructose was replaced with corn starch. Both diets were low in copper. The study had to be terminated when four of the 12 men in the fructose group developed cardiac problems, ranging from severe tachycardia (his heart rate tripled) to mild heart attacks, within the first 11 weeks. This kind of result is why it's easier to get funding for rat studies. The rats don't employ high-quality legal teams so the risk of being bankrupted by doing a fructose study is somewhat minimised. This was the only US study I was able to find where they had actually tried purposefully to feed humans a fructose-based diet. Dr Yudkin had done some similar studies using ordinary table sugar fed to people in UK hospitals, but they were much shorter in duration.

It looked like Surgeon-Captain Cleave might have been on to something. First Dr Yudkin and then the USDA had systematically proven that, at least in rats (and no-one was game to try humans again), it was not a good idea to eat sugar in the quantities found in the American diet in the '80s. And the reason for that was clearly identified as being related to the fructose half of sugar and not the glucose half. The big question for me at this point was why? Why should fructose have all these nasty side effects? What was the body doing with it that created all the problems? And why, given it's been a part of our diet since the dawn of (our) time, was it suddenly a problem? It was time to immerse myself in the chemistry of fructose.

Doctors had known for a long time that diabetic patients could manage their illness by being careful with their diet. By trial and error, doctors knew that some foods produced a sharp increase in blood sugar and others did not. Carbohydrates were divided into simple and complex groups. Diabetics were advised to avoid simple carbohydrates like sugars, white rice and white bread, which were known to increase blood sugar sharply, and seek out complex carbohydrates like wholegrain breads, oats, mueslis and brown rice.

In 1976, Phyllis Crapo, a nutritionist at the University of California in San Diego, published a study that proved that while this advice was generally good, there was one simple carbohydrate that was an exception. Fructose did not affect blood-sugar levels in the same way that other simple carbohydrates did. She went on to show definitively in subsequent studies during the late '70s and early '80s that diabetic patients could be fed fructose without risking increased blood-sugar levels. Based on this research, in 1984 the American Diabetic Association recommended that diabetic patients be given foods that used fructose as the sweetener rather than sugar. Clearly they hadn't been reading about Dr Reiser's rats or they might have reconsidered the advice.

It took a while to sink in, but by 2002 the ADA had completely reversed its recommendation on fructose, saying that added fructose should be completely avoided. They didn't justify their change of heart other than to say that, notwithstanding its proven lack of blood-sugar response, 'fructose may adversely affect plasma lipids'. That's doctor-speak for eating fructose may increase the amount of fat you have circulating in your bloodstream, something Dr Yudkin had been saying since at least the late '70s. Clearly something had given them a big enough scare to make them completely reverse their recommendation on fructose. Perhaps they had finally caught up on their reading and come across some of Dr Reiser's unfortunate rats (and people).

6. BIOCHEMISTRY 101

The thing that was worrying me by now was what happens to all that fructose that we're eating? I was about to discover that the answer (in a nutshell) is that it is turned into fat. And, unlike fat, it bypasses the control mechanisms that we have evolved to stop us eating too much of it. Eating fructose is like eating fat that your body can't detect as being fat.

While Dr Reiser was feeding rats too much fructose, new cell-cloning techniques and gene research were allowing biochemists to figure out exactly how fructose is absorbed by the body and what happens to it after it hits your bloodstream. By 2001, the research of many biochemists over the preceding decade and a half had resulted in the consolidated view that I am about to outline. There may be a drier and more incomprehensible area of science than biochemistry, but so far I haven't come across it. Stay with me though, because as it turns out, the key to all the observations made by doctors Yudkin, Cleave, Reiser and their colleagues is at the cellular level.

The cells of our body cannot just help themselves to blood sugars (glucose, galactose or fructose). They need to have a special protein within the cell itself in order to absorb the sugar and then use it in a chemical process inside the cell. As a family, these proteins are called glucose transporters, or GLUTs for short. Thankfully biochemists are a pragmatic lot and rather than name each of them after their favourite Greek or Latin word, they just numbered each of the GLUTs. I found that the best way to think of a GLUT is that it exposes an indent on the outside of a cell into which only one type of sugar molecule will fit. Sort of like a jigsaw puzzle looking for a missing piece. When a molecule of the right shape comes along, it locks into the molecule-shaped hole made by the GLUT in the cell wall. The GLUT then pushes the sugar through the cell wall and waits for the next molecule to come along.

So far, biochemists have identified 13 different members of the GLUT family. They are not entirely sure what all of them are for, but GLUTs 1 to 5, the important ones from our perspective, are well settled. GLUTs 1, 3 and 4 are for glucose only, GLUT5 is only for fructose, and GLUT2 is for both glucose and fructose.

GLUT1 is used by almost all cells in the body to take up the low levels of glucose required to sustain respiration. It is present in large quantities in foetuses and at much lower levels in adults, where it is concentrated in red blood cells. Its concentration increases when there is less glucose in the blood and decreases when there is more. GLUT1 is the basic 'keep every cell alive' protein, which makes sure our cells are getting enough glucose to keep functioning.

GLUT2 is the protein used by the liver to absorb both glucose and fructose. It is also the glucose sensor used by the islets of Langerhans in the pancreas to determine how much insulin or glucagon to release into the bloodstream. As we shall shortly see, fructose is absorbed through the GLUT2 proteins, but because the pancreatic cells have none of the enzyme needed to use fructose, they are pushed straight back out again. Fructose molecules go whizzing through the GLUT2 proteins without eliciting any response at all and no insulin is produced.

Besides the islets of Langerhans, GLUT2 is also found in the liver and the hypothalamus. GLUT2 is insulin dependent, which means that the number of glucose molecules that it transports across the cell wall (and therefore detects) is regulated by how much insulin is present in the blood. The more insulin there is in the blood, the more glucose GLUT2 transports and the more insulin is produced. Using this simple mechanism, the level of insulin in the blood should always parallel the level of blood sugar in healthy humans.

GLUT3 is the specialist transporter located predominantly in our brains and, to be specific, in the neurons. Like GLUT1, GLUT3 is not dependent on the presence of insulin. It keeps vacuuming glucose out of our blood even if there is no insulin at all. It's a handy design feature shared by all animals, that GLUT1 (for breathing) and GLUT3 (for thinking) keep working even if there is some problem with our energy intake and detection system.

GLUT4 is the really important member of the family for those of us interested in how the body uses and stores energy. GLUT4 is present in large quantities in our muscle and fat tissues and, like GLUT2, it is insulin dependent. The presence of insulin stimulates muscle and fat cells to move all their GLUT4 proteins up to the cell boundary, priming the cell to suck as much glucose as it can out of the blood as fast as possible. This is how insulin stimulates energy use by muscles and fat storage by fat cells. The more insulin there is in the blood, the faster the glucose is vacuumed up by the GLUT4 proteins in the muscles and fat cells.

GLUT5 is the protein associated with the absorption of fructose. You will find GLUT5 in only one place in a healthy female body – the small intestine. In men, it's also present in the testes for reasons that are not entirely clear to biochemists at this stage. In the small intestine, GLUT5 is present in significant quantities. Its only purpose is to vacuum up any fructose we eat and transport it directly from the intestine into our bloodstream. Since the existence of GLUT5 and its role in fructose absorption was first confirmed in 1992, a range of interesting rat tests (yes – everyone is still too scared to test fructose on humans . . . except at the local juice bar) have revealed some intriguing facts about the way we ingest fructose. It seems the amount of GLUT5 present in the intestine is directly related to how much fructose rats (and by extension, humans) eat. Within one day of starting a high-fructose diet, the number of GLUT5 proteins in the rats' intestines had increased fivefold and continued to increase gradually for as long as the fructose diet continued. The body actually manufactures more GLUT5 proteins to make sure we have plenty on hand just in case we encounter some more fructose.

Let's just back up a little here because this is an important point. What the research is telling us is that firstly, we can't absorb fructose through our intestine at all unless we have GLUT5 proteins there. Secondly, the more fructose we eat, the more GLUT5 proteins we make, which means the more fructose we can absorb efficiently. And we're not talking about glacial reaction speeds here. The body reacts immediately and decisively. As soon as fructose is introduced to our gut, the body significantly ramps up our ability to ensure it enters our bloodstream. It's almost as if we are designed to detect and absorb as much fructose as we can possibly get our hands on as fast as possible. If fructose is present in our food, we don't want to waste one gram of it.

Apparently age also makes a difference to the number of GLUT5 proteins we have available. Rats and rabbits have no significant

Protein	Transports . . .	Stimulated by . . .	Location	Purpose
GLUT1	Glucose	Works all the time	Every cell	Keeps every cell alive
GLUT2	Glucose and fructose	The amount of insulin in the blood	Pancreas, hypothalamus and liver	Detects the presence of glucose
GLUT3	Glucose	Works all the time	Brain	Keeps the brain alive
GLUT4	Glucose	The amount of insulin in the blood	Fat and muscles	Powers the muscles and stores glucose as fat
GLUT5	Fructose	The amount of fructose ingested	Small intestine	Gets as much fructose into our bloodstream as possible

Figure 6.1: The GLUT proteins and their uses.

quantities of GLUT5 until after they are weaned. Human children one to three years of age on normal diets (don't worry, no-one was feeding children fructose to see what happened) also seem to lack it in significant quantities. The symptoms of a lack of GLUT5 are exactly the same as those of an inability to absorb lactose . . . abdominal pain and chronic non-specific diarrhoea (often called toddler's diarrhoea). A series of studies conducted in 1996 appeared to link the lack of development of GLUT5 with these symptoms in most toddlers. So it seems toddlers have a built-in resistance to fructose in the diet. The results of over-consumption might not be too pretty on the outside, but on the inside of their little bodies, fructose is not getting into the bloodstream. By the time you finish reading the next section, you'll wish you were still a toddler.

GLUT5 is not present in significant quantities anywhere in our body except in the intestine. This makes it quite different from the first four GLUTs, which deal with glucose. Glucose is sucked out of our bloodstream by the first four GLUTs and distributed all over our body. The only place after digestion that contains GLUT5 (and therefore an ability to use fructose) is the testes. In a healthy body, no other cell has any use for all the fructose being vacuumed up by the GLUT5 in our intestine. Even the testes have only a very limited capacity to absorb it. The location and function of GLUT5 explains Dr Crapo's observation in the '70s that fructose did not cause insulin levels in the blood to increase, but perhaps the American Diabetics Association (ADA) should have dug a little deeper before recommending that every diabetic pig out on fructose.

Some interesting research published in 1996 by the Sloan-Kettering Cancer Center in New York showed that very high levels of GLUT5 were also found in the breast tissue of women suffering from breast cancer. Normally GLUT5 is not found in breast tissue at all. Not surprisingly, the presence of GLUT5 in breast tissue is now being studied as a potential early-detection test for breast cancer. The folks conducting the Molecular Imaging Program at Stanford University confirmed the viability of just such a test in 2008. Obviously, there is a difference between GLUT5 distribution in healthy bodies as opposed to the bodies of people suffering from some diseases.

So if, when we are healthy, none of our cells except those in the liver has any significant ability to use fructose, what on earth are our bodies doing with all that fructose that we are so efficiently absorbing from our food?

To answer that question it looked like I needed to come to grips with what was going on in the liver, and to do that I needed to understand a biochemical process called glycolysis (from the Greek *glyc* – sweet; *lysis* – letting loose). Unfortunately, Latin and Greek seemed to be the preferred naming conventions for biochemists after a brief bout with being logical in simply numbering the GLUT proteins.

So far I have been saying that glucose is used by our cells to produce energy that keeps us upright and breathing. The role of glucose in keeping us alive was observed by some of the very earliest biochemists; all of them wanted to know how exactly that trick was achieved. One of the phrases I came across a lot when reading about the history of the discoveries in carbohydrate metabolism was 'the process was turning out to be much more complex than had been imagined 10 years before'. It was a phrase I was beginning to sympathise with wholeheartedly, the more I read in this area.

One of the pioneers of human metabolic biochemistry was an English chap by the name of Arthur Harden. Born in Manchester in 1865, in 1912 he took up a professorship in Biochemistry at the University of London, where he stayed until his retirement in 1930, one year after he collected the Nobel Prize in Chemistry. The Nobel

Prize was for a paper he wrote in 1906 that described how phosphate is used by yeast cells to convert glucose to ethanol and carbon dioxide. This process, known as fermentation (yep, the same one used in making beer and wine), is the means by which some chemicals seem to be able to cause carbohydrates first to decompose, and then to transform themselves into other substances altogether.

In 1897, German chemist Eduard Buchner had proved that extracts of yeast that definitively contained no living organisms (because he pulverised the yeast with a mortar and pestle before using it) were able to turn sugar into alcohol and carbon dioxide – something the wine industry had known at a practical level for millennia – by adding phosphates. This proved that a chemical substance rather than a living organism in the yeast was responsible for the fermentation. Buchner had called the substance zymase, but we know these substances today as enzymes. Buchner picked up the 1907 Nobel Prize in Chemistry for this discovery.

In his fermentation experiments, Harden managed to separate out the zymase from the rest of the yeast mixture produced according to Buchner's recipe. He proved that the zymase was in fact the thing that powered the fermenting. Without the zymase, the yeast was inert – nothing interesting happened no matter how much phosphate you added to it. If, however, phosphate and the enzyme were present, fermentation would proceed until all of the glucose was used up. The relevance of that observation wasn't immediately obvious, but it is credited with being the foundation stone of an important new branch of biochemistry, intermediary metabolism. This branch concentrates on the study of compounds that come into existence, often only very briefly, during the course of many biochemical reactions.

Harden had found that an enzyme was critical to the chemical process called fermentation, which our bodies used to turn glucose into energy, but things were still a little misty beyond that. In 1936, the same year Harden was knighted for his work, Herman Kalckar, a Danish biochemist, confirmed the central role of an energy-carrying molecule in the fermentation process described by Harden. Kalckar proved by studying frog legs that phosphate compounds did produce energy. It's a pity he wasn't French or I could have come up with all manner of amusing double entendres at this point. He proved that he could get the muscles in frog legs to continue to contract using phosphates, even when they were cut off (literally) from their normal sources of energy.

In 1941, Kalckar's collaborator, Fritz Lipmann, confirmed the existence of ATP (adenosine triphosphate). Lipmann was a German biochemist who received the Nobel Prize in Medicine for his discovery in 1945 of an enzyme critical to the oxidation of fatty acids (the way our body converts fat to energy). More important to our discussion at the moment, however, is his confirmation of the existence of ATP.

ATP is the energy highway of our body; it stores and transports energy. The glucose that is dragged into our cells through the GLUT receptors is converted into ATP by a chemical reaction involving phosphates and an enzyme. To release the energy, just add water and another enzyme. If an enzyme is present, water reacts with the ATP to produce energy, another chemical called ADP (adenosine diphosphate) and a phosphate. Every single day every one of us creates and destroys an amount of ATP equivalent to our own body weight. The energy released by that series of reactions is how we convert glucose into energy and what keeps us powered up. That series of reactions is what biochemists call glycolysis.

As Harden first proved, glycolysis does not happen unless the enzymes are present. This means that controlling the enzymes is a way to throttle the process, and it turns out this is exactly what the body does with its hormones. The hormones discussed earlier, in particular insulin and glucagon, activate or shut down these enzyme switches in our cells by shuffling the enzyme molecules between the nucleus (where they are hidden from view) and the cell boundary (where they can do their stuff).

The exact chemistry of how ATP is produced and used by our cells had to wait until the '80s and '90s and is still subject to ongoing study (the 1997 Nobel Prize in Chemistry went to folks studying ATP) – as I said at the start of this section and many have said before me, it always turns out to be more complex than we thought 10 years ago. Some of the more recent investigations have, however, shed some light on differences between how glucose and fructose are treated in the process of glycolysis. These differences pretty solidly explain much of what doctors Yudkin and Reiser saw happening to the rats they fed too much fructose in the '60s and '70s.

Remember that in order for the whole glycolysis process to keep going the cells need a good supply of the right enzymes. As the good Dr Harden found, no enzyme means no reaction and no energy. We have four enzymes used for converting blood sugars into energy. One is a general-purpose enzyme that is available in pretty much every cell in our body, and the other three are specialist enzymes (one for each type of sugar) that are found only in our liver.

Hexokinase is the name of the general-purpose sugar-converting enzyme; 'hexo' because all three sugars have molecules that look like hexagons. Hexokinase is distributed throughout the body and theoretically could be used to convert all three sugars into energy, but it doesn't convert anything other than glucose. Even though our cells could use hexokinase to convert all that circulating fructose into energy, they don't get the chance because hexokinase can only

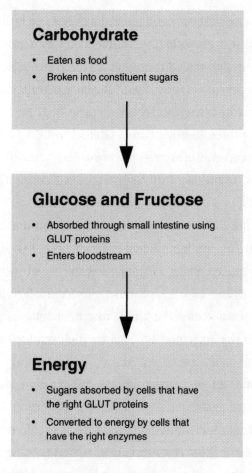

Figure 6.2: How carbohydrates end up being turned into energy.

be used to convert whatever sugar actually gets inside the cell. Most of the healthy cells in our body do not possess the GLUT (GLUT2 or GLUT5) proteins necessary to suck fructose through the cell wall. All they have is ordinary old garden variety GLUT1, which only vacuums up glucose. GLUT1 and hexokinase provide our underlying 'power on' state for all cells, and GLUT3 does the same thing for the brain. Fat cells also have plenty of hexokinase but, instead of GLUT1, they have GLUT4 proteins, so they also only work on glucose.

There's a pecking order at the blood glucose buffet. Brain cells and ordinary cells get to eat first. Their GLUT protein works whether there is insulin or not and they have an enzyme ready to convert the glucose they get into energy just to stay alive. Then, as insulin levels increase, fat and muscle cells get to dine because insulin triggers their GLUT proteins. But neither GLUT1, GLUT3 (the brain) nor GLUT4 (fat and muscle) proteins are able to absorb fructose. The fructose goes sailing merrily by most of our cells – that is, until it gets to the liver.

Things are different in the liver. Liver cells are full of GLUT2 proteins that can absorb glucose *and* fructose. Just like GLUT4 in the fat and muscle cells, GLUT2 is sensitive to insulin. As insulin levels rise, the GLUT2 proteins suck more and more glucose and fructose into liver cells. That's where we find the three specialist enzymes. The enzyme needed to use glucose is (not illogically) called glucokinase ('ase' being the ending meaning enzyme). The one used for fructose is fructokinase and, you guessed it, galactokinase is for galactose.

The primary function of glucokinase is to convert excess blood sugar into our temporary short-term batteries (glycogen) and our longer-term energy stores (fatty acids). Unlike hexokinase, glucokinase is not active all the time. At normal pre-meal concentrations of blood sugar, the liver is a net producer of glucose (using up the batteries to keep us humming along). It's only when blood glucose and insulin start to rise after a meal that the liver starts to access the glucose in the bloodstream, using glucokinase, to create short-term energy storage, the backup energy it had been using before you ate that doughnut. Glucokinase needs insulin in order to function, and glucokinase itself is less efficient than hexokinase. These two facts together put the liver third in line at the blood sugar buffet.

Brain cells and normal cells will take glucose if it's there and use it immediately. Fat and muscle cells must wait until insulin kicks in but once it does they can compete equally with the other cells. Liver cells also have to wait for insulin but have a less powerful enzyme, which slows down their use of the glucose.

Under normal conditions, the vast majority of the glucose absorbed by the liver is converted to glycogen for storage, plus a little energy to keep the whole mechanism working. If too much energy is created, a secondary process converts the excess into fatty acids, which are pumped out into our bloodstream.

There is normally very little fatty acid production, because there is a very important control point in the whole process. So far, in an effort to keep the process of glycolysis even remotely explainable, I've combined a lot of steps together; however, at this point it's necessary to dive a little deeper.

Around the middle of the progression from glucose to energy, Dr Kalckar's energy-transport molecule, ATP, is created. The enzyme used to create it is called (wait for it) phosphofructokinase-1 (PFK-1). PFK-1 is a gatekeeper that stops the liver making too much energy and fat. It creates ATP (which eventually turns into energy if needed, with any leftovers being turned into fat), but if there is too much ATP in the cell, PFK-1 is deactivated. If ATP is being used up quickly, then there will be relatively little of it in the cell and PFK-1 will be switched on to make some more. It's a very simple and elegant feedback mechanism that means that, in normal conditions, we are designed not to make too much energy and therefore not to create excess circulating fatty acids out of the leftovers.

GLUT2 proteins in the liver are just as good at sucking fructose into the cells as they are at vacuuming up glucose. At last, circulating fructose has found some cells that are happy to invite them inside. And once they get through the door, they find fructokinase waiting with open arms. Fructokinase does not need insulin to start going to work on fructose. It starts converting it to ATP immediately and rapidly. Very rapidly, in fact. Fructose can be absorbed by the liver twice as fast as glucose and it gets a significant head start as well, because it doesn't have to wait for insulin to fire it up. With fructose in the blood, the liver can elbow its way to the head of the buffet line.

The gut will process as much fructose as we put in our mouths, with no known limit. The liver has no competition for the fructose in the blood. It's the only major organ with the GLUT protein needed to drag it out of the bloodstream *and* the enzyme needed to convert it to energy. It doesn't have to wait for insulin levels to rise before it can get started on the main course, and it can eat it up twice as fast as it can eat glucose. Sounds like a pretty efficient way to get energy – eating fructose is kind of like throwing on the afterburners.

There's just one little problem: it is a very small detail, but it might just be the detail that lies behind a significant number of our modern health problems, including the obesity epidemic. When fructokinase creates ATP, it bypasses the step in the glycolysis process that is controlled by PFK-1. Remember, the PFK-1 enzyme stops us getting fat on glucose. When too much ATP is produced, PFK-1 switches off and stops the process. As Harden found, no enzyme means no chemical reaction. Fructose skips that critical regulatory step. It jumps straight to ATP with no regulation at all. If we have lots of fructose in our blood, it automatically and rapidly overloads the ATP production system of the liver. Our ever-efficient bodies don't waste all that ATP; it just gets converted straight to fatty acids.

Small quantities of fructose don't have any serious effects. A little extra ATP is created, which shuts down the glucose absorption until ATP levels return to normal. But put a lot of fructose into that loop and it doesn't matter how long the glucose system is shut down for; fructose will still keep pumping up the ATP volume and the fat production. That one little detail – that fructose bypasses the glycolysis control mechanism in the liver – means that it directly creates vast amounts of circulating fatty acids (including LDL cholesterol).

Interesting research in 2003 by scientists from the Department of Molecular Physiology and Biophysics at the Vanderbilt University in Nashville, Tennessee, showed that fructose has exactly the same stimulatory effect on glucokinase as insulin. Biochemists now believe that a small amount of fructose in the diet is necessary to get the glucose processing under way. Small amounts of fructose appear to be a sort of starter motor for our glucose digestion in the liver. The fructose acts to stimulate the glucokinase activity in anticipation of the release of insulin by the pancreas. So we need a little fructose in our daily diet – probably about the same amount as you would find in a couple of pieces of fruit. From an evolutionary perspective, this probably makes sense, since prior to about 1830 that was just about the only way to get fructose into your tummy.

Fructose also skips the glucose-driven control mechanisms of the pancreas. If we consume more fructose each day than what is found in one or two pieces of fruit, it is ignored by the pancreas and no insulin is released in response to its consumption. This was the big discovery that inspired the ADA to decree fructose as the preferred sweetener for diabetics. Biochemistry has since caught up with observation and we now clearly understand why this is so. Like the liver, the pancreas uses GLUT2 transporters to absorb both glucose and fructose. Unlike the liver, the pancreas has almost no fructokinase, which means that although the fructose is transported into the cell, it can't be used so it is washed straight back out again. That, on its own, would be nothing to worry about. It's what's going on in the liver that's the dangerous part. Fructose is being efficiently converted to fat faster than you can say phosphofructokinase. Telling diabetics (or anyone else) to eat pure fructose was, and is, an exceedingly dangerous thing to do.

Back to the question that started my hunt through the arcane world of molecular biochemistry – what happens to all that fructose? The answer appears to be this: it gets rapidly and totally converted to circulating fatty acids and manages to avoid all of our control mechanisms in the process. When we eat carbohydrates, proteins and fat, insulin and CCK tell us when to stop eating, and insulin and PFK-1 control the use of the glucose. There are no equivalent controls for fructose.

When the only fructose in our diet was in ripe fruit, this didn't matter much. We have enough fructose sensors in our pancreas to trigger an insulin response in the quantities found in a few pieces of fruit. It is only when we over-consume fructose that the 'loophole' in our appetite-control mechanism opens up. In a modern diet, where most food is now flavoured with fructose compounds (like sugar and high-fructose corn syrup), this is a recipe for obesity and much worse.

As far as our pancreas is concerned, fructose calories are largely invisible. Insulin release is not triggered by its consumption. Earlier I described the GI diets, which became popular in the last decade. You'll remember that the theory behind a GI diet (for people who aren't diabetic) is that, because the food has a low GI, insulin is not

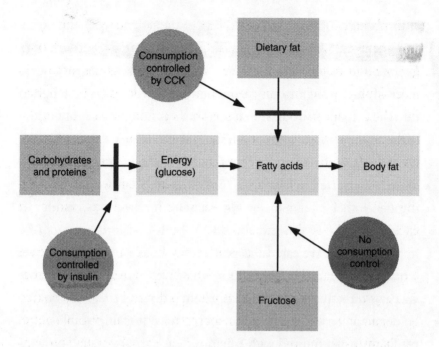

Figure 6.3: The fructose loophole in our appetite-control system.

released and fat storage is inhibited. Insulin is, however, only used for converting glucose into fat. It is not required to convert circulating fatty acids into fat. If we eat a high-fructose diet, the fructose will be converted directly to fatty acids and, in turn, body fat. Given the choice, our fat cells would much rather store circulating fatty acids as fat than go to all the trouble of converting glucose to body fat using insulin. It only takes 2.5 calories to convert 100 calories of fatty acids into body fat. It takes 23 calories (10 times as much energy) to convert 100 calories of protein or glucose into body fat. So, given the choice, our bodies will store fatty acids every time, that being the more energy-efficient course to follow.

That's a lot of biochemical mumbo jumbo to absorb in one sitting, so let's recap. We have one primary appetite-control centre in our brain called the hypothalamus. It reacts to four major appetite hormones. Three of them (insulin, leptin and CCK) tell us when we have had enough to eat, and one of them (ghrelin) temporarily inhibits the effect of the other three and tells us that we need to eat. Every piece of food we consume stimulates the release of one or more of the 'enough to eat' hormones once we have had enough to eat. There is one substance that does not stimulate the release of any of the 'enough to eat' hormones. That substance is fructose. Fructose skips the fat-creation control mechanism in the liver (PFK-1) and is directly converted to fatty acids (and then body fat) without passing through either of our major appetite-control gateways (insulin or CCK). Fructose is also invisible to our built-in calorie counter (the hypothalamus). We can eat as much fructose as we can shove down our throats and never feel full for long. Every gram of the fructose we eat is directly converted to fat. There is no mystery to the obesity epidemic when you know those simple facts. It is impossible not to get fat on a diet infused with fructose.

7. HONEY WITHOUT BEES

The message from the accumulation of all the research I had been reading was clear – fructose bypasses all of our appetite-control systems and jumps a critical step in our metabolism that would ordinarily stop our arteries filling up with circulating fat. Eating fat still puts fat in our arteries, but we have a built-in control to stop us eating too much fat. No such control exists for fructose.

I could see that eating fructose could be really bad news. But how much fructose were we actually eating? Surgeon-Captain Cleave's graph certainly suggested we were eating a lot more sugar than at the turn of the century, and sugar is half fructose. But his graph only went up to 1955. I decided to find out more about whether fructose was really a factor in the modern diet.

Most of the rat studies I read about had used fairly large doses of fructose to produce the results they did. After reading many newspaper articles about medical 'discoveries', I had come to the conclusion you could induce cancer in a rat by feeding it just about anything in a large enough dose. Were we really eating that much fructose?

As we know, fructose is what makes fruit sweet. It's no coincidence that the most popular fruits today are the sweetest-tasting ones. They are also the ones highest in fructose.

So fruit and vegetables are a source of fructose, but not a very rich source. Even the sweetest fruit (the humble apple) contains less than 8 per cent fructose by weight. Put another way, the average apple contains about the same amount of fructose as 2 teaspoons of sugar. The US Department of Agriculture has kept detailed statistics on total US fruit and vegetable consumption since 1970, and the limited statistics available in Australia show similar trends – an increase in consumption, driven largely by an industry that has only really existed since the 1940s, the packaged juice business.

In 1869, a New Jersey dentist and communion steward at his local church, Thomas Welch, successfully applied Louis Pasteur's principles of pasteurisation (discovered just seven years earlier) to

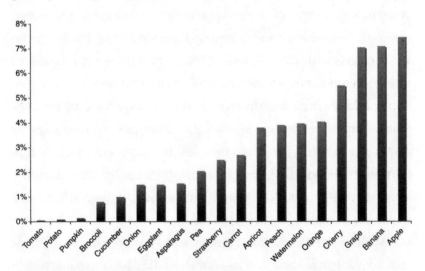

Figure 7.1: The average fructose content by weight of popular fresh fruits and vegetables, based on quantities measured by the USDA.

grape juice. Pasteurisation involves heating liquids just enough to kill most micro-organisms but not so much as to sterilise them by boiling, which usually destroys the taste as well. Until that point the only way to enjoy grape juice was to be there as it was stomped out of the grapes or wait a few years and enjoy the fermented variety that came in a bottle with a cork. Dr Welch had a strong motivation for his work. His invention meant that he didn't have to freshly squeeze the grapes every communion Sunday. Dr Welch's son Charles (also a dentist) decided there was more potential in the production of grape juice than supplying the local altar. After rave reviews from the juice-sipping public at the Chicago World's Fair in 1893, Charles threw in his dental practice and concentrated on the juice business full time.

For some reason, the US government thought their sailors might be more effective warriors if they weren't drunk, so when the US Navy substituted grape juice for wine on all its vessels in 1914, the grape juice industry came into its own. People had tried pasteurising all sorts of other fruit and vegetable juices with no success, but by 1927, the Welch Juice Company was able to extend the methods to tomatoes, and the first non-grape juice rolled off the production lines. Meanwhile, in Evanston, Illinois, WG Peacock applied the Welch pasteurisation methods to a range of vegetables, creating the Vege-Min line of juices, but they were not exactly flying off the shelves until he decided in 1933 to combine eight of them into a drink he called Vege-Min 8. Vege-Min 8 didn't taste great but, at the suggestion of a local grocer, he changed the name to V-8 Juice, added some sugar and increased the amount of tomato juice in the mix. Sales of the new V-8 drink, which was almost 90 per cent tomato juice, really took off in 1936.

Meanwhile, over in California, the methods used to produce tomato juice were being applied to a potentially vastly more lucrative fruit crop, the orange. By the early 1940s, large-scale commercial production of packaged orange juice was possible and the juicing industry has not looked back. Since then, vegetable- and fruit-juice consumption has risen steadily. From a base of zero in 1940, the average US citizen was consuming 43L of fruit juice every year by 2002. The average Australian consumed a more moderate 35L per person per year, but it had nevertheless become a significant addition to the modern diet. And that was before the advent of the modern-day 'juice bar', which has increased Australian fruit juice sales by over 60 per cent from 2003 to 2007. Vegetable juice consumption grew even more rapidly. From a standing start in 1933, Americans were gulping down 81L of vegetable (90 per cent tomato) juice per annum by 2005.

Juicing converts fruit and vegetables from a food source containing significant fibre mass, flavoured with fructose, to one containing little other than fructose and water – oh, and some vitamin C.

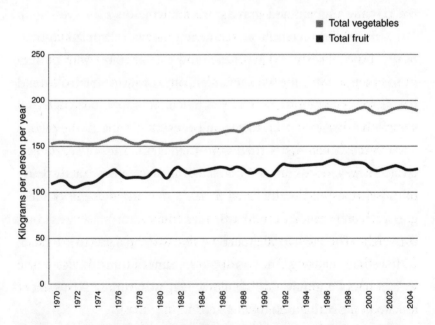

Figure 7.2: Total US fruit and vegetable consumption 1970–2005 – based on USDA data – most of which relates to accelerating consumption of juices.

While our use of fruit and vegetables has increased slightly overall, it has been due largely to increased juice consumption against a background of falling whole fruit and vegetable consumption. We are applying our intellectual and industrial muscle to make sure we extract the sweetness from the food and then throw the rest away. Monkeys on the plains of Africa would do the same if they could, but there is nowhere to plug in their juicing machines. We have, in the last 60 years or so, become very good at getting just the bit we are really interested in and discarding the rest.

Increasing juice consumption is certainly increasing the rate of fructose consumption, but it is by no means the major source of this dangerous substance in the modern diet. Long ago, our ingenious forebears figured out an even more efficient way to extract sweetness from plants, store it and then add it to all of our food. Why hunt for ripe apples and bananas to put in your juicer, when you could make anything as sweet as you wanted?

About 9000 years ago, just as the Egyptians were thinking seriously about odd-shaped buildings and the Chinese were putting in the groundwork for the fireworks that would be needed for the Year 2000 celebrations, some folks in Papua New Guinea detected something that would ultimately affect every person on the planet. They noticed that one of the native grasses was very sweet-tasting. In fact, it was more than twice as sweet as the nearest fruit available to those tribespeople, the banana. Modern analysis reveals that the grass, which grows 2 to 6 metres tall, contains 15 per cent fructose by weight. The Papuan highlanders didn't take the discovery much further than realising that sucking on a sugarcane stem was a nice way to pass the monsoon, but slowly, sugarcane gained popularity as a good thing to have growing around the village.

We now know that once refined and concentrated, sugar is more than six times as sweet as an apple, the sweetest commonly occurring fruit. Refined sugar's 50 per cent fructose content, combined with our lust for sweetness, ensured that sugarcane became one of our earliest successful experiments in cultivation. Over the next 2000 years, its fame slowly spread from island to island, finally making its way to the outer arms of the Hindu empires of Indonesia, from where it swiftly leapt to India. While there was always a ready market for the sweet grass, it was hard to transport without it going bad (it was, after all, just grass – imagine what your grass clippings would look like after a few months at sea), so you had to live in its native tropics to benefit. About seven millennia ago, some folks in India figured out that crushing the stems of the giant grass produced a very sweet 'juice'. Its sap is pure sucrose (table sugar) dissolved in water. The sap was a delicacy used much like honey (and often in place of it) to sweeten foods. When the greatest Greek general of all time, Alexander the Great, conquered the Punjab in 327 BCE, his troops brought the secret of the reed that produced 'honey without bees' back to their Mediterranean homeland. They called it *sakchar*.

By the year 300 our Indian friends had discovered that if they dried the sap, they were left with a very tasty crystal that could be added to any food to make it sweet. Even more importantly, dried sugar crystals lasted much better than cane or sap on long sea voyages. Programmed as we are for sweetness, cultivating sugarcane naturally became a very high priority and crystallised sugar suddenly became a valuable and highly tradable 'spice'.

By 540, the Persians (modern-day Iranians) had learned the Indian secrets of making *sakchar*. Not unsurprisingly, the Arabians decided that sugar production was a skill that was worth copying when their armies conquered Persia in 641. The Arabian armies took the secrets with them so when they invaded Sicily in 800, one of the first crops to be planted was sugarcane. Sugar mills were set up and a brisk trade in the white gold was established all across the Arabian lands. When the Christian crusades rolled through the holy lands at the beginning of the second millennium, one of the treasures they took back to England was the secret of sugar.

In England, for many centuries, sugar was an expensive commodity. Nevertheless, demand for sugar was irrepressible. By 1259 it was readily available if you had the money (the equivalent of $285 per kilo). Sugar certainly wasn't cheap but, if you had the cash, there was plenty you could do with it. Culinary discoveries flooded in from the Americas in the 1400s and 1500s. Coffee, tea and chocolate were all bitter on their own, but add a little sugar and, voilà, suddenly you have luxurious new treats. Only 15 per cent of soup recipes in cookbooks from the 1500s included sweet ingredients, and those that did mostly added honey. But the incessant demand for sugar made it profitable to bring more and more of the product into the market, which in turn drove the price down. By the 1800s almost half of all published soup recipes were sweetened.

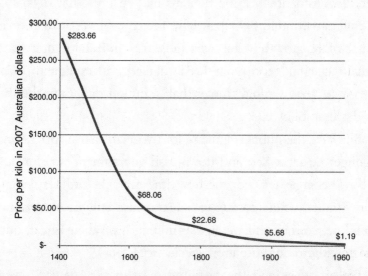

Figure 7.3: English retail price of sugar 1400–1960 in 2007 Australian dollars – no wonder it was described as 'white gold' in the 1400s.

In 1400, sugar was still way too expensive for the average peasant on the street, but the price was coming down quickly as England's empire expanded to include tropical lands where sugarcane grew in natural abundance. By the middle of the 15th century there were plantations in Madeira, the Canary Islands and St Thomas, supplying Europe with sugar. By the end of the 16th century, sugar farming and milling had spread over the greater part of tropical America, followed in the next century by the development of sugar exports from the West Indies. The demand for sugar was one of the major reasons for the slave trade for two centuries or more – cutting down 5-metre-high cane fields requires a lot of very cheap labour.

Britain took Jamaica and other parts of the West Indies from Spain in 1655 and from then on became heavily involved in the sugar industry. By 1750 there were 120 sugar refineries operating in Britain. Their combined annual output was still only 30 000 tons but the enormous demand ensured sugar was extremely profitable. Profitable commodities attract the tax man like moths to a flame. Every government since the Romans had ensured that sugar filled the coffers with gold (which is why, today, we have such excellent records of the growth of the sugar industry). In Britain, for instance, annual sugar tax receipts in 1781 totalled $50 million in today's terms, and grew tenfold to over half a billion dollars in the three decades that followed.

By 1874, the public's demand for reasonable sugar prices could no longer be repressed and the British government was forced to abolish the sugar tax. For the first time ever, the ordinary citizens of the Empire could afford to eat sugar (it was still the equivalent of $25 a kilo, so they still weren't sprinkling it on their cereal, but at least now they could use it on special occasions).

Lower prices and the resulting mass-market demand meant that industrial-scale production could accelerate. Many of today's taken-for-granted foods such as confectionery, cakes and biscuits, as well as sweetened drinks, were invented and popularised towards the end of the nineteenth century around sugar as a major ingredient (which by then cost 'just' $7 a kilo).

Prussia (a region located approximately in modern-day Germany) was not terribly happy about the state of affairs in the sugarcane trade. It didn't own any tropical territories to speak of and this meant that if Prussians wanted sugar (and they did, of course), they had to buy it from one of their European cousins after paying a suitable 'tax'. This was intermittently complicated by being at war with said cousins. The Prussians decided they needed an alternative to sugarcane that could be grown in nice handy places like, say, northern Europe, rather than having to travel to irritatingly hot places, controlled by enemies of the state, just to get some sugar in their coffee. Prussian scientists were immediately set the task of testing all available northern European plants to find a replacement for sugarcane.

In 1747, Franz Achard succeeded in identifying the beet species as the one with the maximum sugar content. By the start of the nineteenth century, German sugar beet crops began delivering good enough yields to allow European-grown plants to compete with imported sugarcane as a source of the 'white gold'. Nelson's victory at Trafalgar in 1805 and the ensuing naval blockade of Europe guaranteed that sugar beet became the source of sugar for continental Europe from then on. By 1860, such was the demand for sugar that Germany changed from being a net importer of sugar to an exporter.

In the United States, sugarcane cultivation began in the tropical climate of New Orleans in the eighteenth century. Early attempts to create a sugar industry in the United States did not fare well. From the late 1830s, when the first factory was built, until the 1870s, sugar factories closed down almost as quickly as they opened. And attempts to create a home-grown sugar industry weren't helped by the destruction of the sugar industry in the Gulf states during the US Civil War. Finally, in 1872, a Californian factory was able profitably to produce sugar in significant quantities. After that shaky start, the US sugar industry grew at breakneck speed. At the dawn of the twentieth century, more than 30 factories were in operation in the United States.

Sugar arrived in Australia with the first convicts in 1788. The First Fleet picked up some sugarcane on the way past South Africa and planted the first crop at Port Macquarie. As with the rest of the world, actually producing sugar in commercial quantities proved difficult until the first viable mill got going at Hastings, New South Wales, in 1867. By 1868, there were nine mills producing 60 tons of sugar a year in New South Wales. The by then separate colony of Queensland produced 30 tons of sugar that year. By 1885, there were 102 mills in New South Wales and 166 in Queensland. Queensland had the advantage of cheap (virtually free) indentured labour from Polynesia to work the plantations. By 1924, Australia was producing more sugar than it could consume and exporting commenced. By the end of World War II, Australia was producing 950 000 tons per annum. By 1954, it was 1.3 million tons and by 1980 this had more than doubled again to 3 million tonnes. By 2000, Australia was producing more than 4.6 million tonnes (worth $1.2 billion) of sugar a year. Today, 85 per cent of Australia's sugar crop is exported, making Australia the second-largest sugar exporter in the world, behind Brazil.

Everybody really liked the sweet stuff. Demand for sugar grew more quickly than even the exponential growth in world population. In the 1830s, when the world population had just passed 1 billion, sugar production was about 800g per year for every person in the world. By the mid-1970s, with the population standing at just over 4 billion, world sugar production stood at 20kg for every man, woman and child on the planet. People were by then consuming 25 times as much sugar as their great-granddaddy had just 140 years earlier.

The injection of cane (and eventually beet) sugar into the western diet introduced a significant new source of fructose for the first time in the evolutionary history of humans. At the start of the nineteenth century, annual average fructose consumption was less than a kilo a year, sourced almost entirely from eating fresh fruit, and honey for the occasional treat (honey was neither cheap nor plentiful). By 1885, every adult over the age of 20 in the United States was consuming 13kg of added fructose in the form of 25kg of sugar, a substance that their parents had never even seen, let alone tasted.

By 1909 US sugar consumption had almost doubled again to nearly 40kg per person per year, and by the early 1930s, Americans were eating almost 50kg of sugar per year. And that's where our fructose consumption probably would have stayed had it not been for the invention of some interesting new ways to add fructose to our diet. From 1930 to 1970, sugar consumption plateaued at just under 50kg per year (except for some rationing caused by World War II, which saw consumption fall). Obviously we had added sugar to just about everything that we wanted sweetened. There seemed to be a natural limit to how sweet we wanted our food to be. Price was no longer the issue. At less than $1 per kilo, anybody could afford to eat nothing but sugar if they wanted to. Clearly (as any mother of an engorged two-year-old will tell you) you can eat only so many lollies, biscuits and cakes before you get sick.

If you had wanted a cool drink on a hot summer's day in 1886 in downtown Atlanta, Georgia, you wouldn't have had many options. The introduction of prohibition earlier in the year meant that beer and anything harder was out. So you might have been tempted to wander into Jacob's Pharmacy (the largest in town) and head for the soda fountain for a long glass of carbonated water, what we call soda water today. Soda water was considered to be beneficial to general wellbeing and soda fountains had become very popular. That summer, for the first time ever, you would also have been able to buy (for the grand sum of 5 cents – $1.30 in 2007 Australian dollars), a glass of Dr Pemberton's French Wine Coca, a nerve tonic, stimulant and headache remedy. The Coca was a syrupy sweet brown liquid that had a tangy taste reminiscent of caramel and vanilla, with a little kick from the crushed leaves of the coca plant (perhaps more famous today for its other product, nose candy) and caffeine-rich kola nuts. About six months later, an enterprising soda jerk decided to jazz up his soda water by adding Dr Pemberton's syrup to the glass. Coca-Cola was born. Ten litres of Coca-Cola syrup was made by mixing up 1.4kg of sugar with 7.5L of water and a series of secret flavouring ingredients that included caramel, vanilla, coca leaves and kola nuts. Today, 1.2 billion serves of it are sold every year.

Coca-Cola – today consisting essentially of sugar, flavouring and carbonated water – was one of the first flavoured 'soft' drink concoctions, but it was by no means the only one. By the turn of the twentieth century, there were over a hundred different brands of carbonated soft drink on sale in the United States, with the most popular flavour being ginger ale.

Turning the flavoured syrup into the fizzy drink we know today was simply a matter of adding five parts soda water to one part syrup. It was a recipe that lent itself to very efficient distribution. Instead of shipping the end product around the country, pharmacies and (by 1889) bottlers could be sent barrels of syrup that they could mix with water for local sales. Bottled soft drinks were immediately popular with the buying public – now they could take them home and enjoy their favourite 'soda' any time they wished – but it was not until 1928 that bottle sales outstripped soda fountain sales.

By the end of World War II, the average American was drinking 38L of carbonated soft drink every year. That alone accounted for 4 of the 44kg (9 per cent) of sugar they were then consuming every year. Two decades later, in 1965, they were drinking twice as much soft drink and it accounted for 8 of the 44kg (18 per cent) of sugar they were consuming every year. Liquid sugar was quickly replacing confectionery as the primary source of sugar in the American diet. By 1985, soft-drink consumption had doubled again, but the availability of new low-calorie sugar substitutes meant that only three-quarters of the drinks sold were 'full strength'.

Soaring world sugar prices and a plummeting market for corn during the 1960s and '70s drove the US corn industry to invest heavily in promising research focused on converting cornstarch-derived glucose into the much sweeter, and therefore more valuable, fructose. In 1968, the first commercial shipment of high-fructose corn syrup (HFCS) capable of being used as a sugar substitute hit the market. In just two decades it displaced cane sugar as America's primary source of fructose. Today 42 per cent of all corn grown in the United States goes into the manufacture of HFCS. This has occurred in no small measure because the makers of Coke and Pepsi, who between them purchased almost 20 per cent of all sugar sold in the United States at the time, decided to switch from sugar to HFCS in the early 1980s. The relatively low cost of HFCS enabled food companies to 'super-size' food portions, particularly drinks, at little cost, increasing profits and perceived value for customers. HFCS fast became the primary sweetener for manufactured food products in the United States.

By 1985, Americans were consuming 16kg of sugar (or HFCS) from soft drink every single year. Total sugar and HFCS consumption was only slightly higher, at 46kg, but full-strength soft drink now represented 35 per cent of the sugar the average American consumed in a year. By the turn of the century, Americans were consuming 26kg of HFCS in soft drinks, but by now America had moved off the sweetness plateau and total sugar consumption had also increased. Nevertheless, soft drinks still represented 44 per cent of the 60kg of sugar consumed by the average American in a year.

In 1870, the only way anyone could eat any significant amount of fructose was either to be the king of England (or a close relative), or to come into the small fortune required to buy sugar or honey. Alternatively, you could buy a lot of fruit and juice it yourself. Whichever way you cut it, money was required. There was no cheap or easy way to eat fructose in any kind of quantity. But 130 years later, the average American was eating 33kg of fructose every

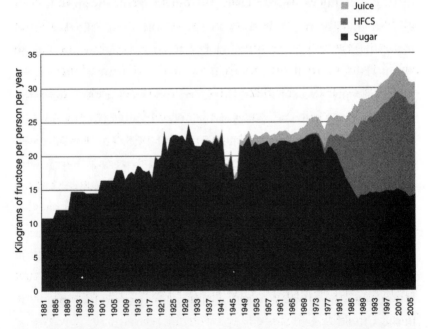

Figure 7.4: Total per capita US fructose consumption by source – the amount of added fructose went from nothing in 1870 to over 30kg per year by the year 2000.

single year just from sugar, HFCS and fruit juices. And that was before you started counting consumption from honey and syrups (together a further kilo per annum).

Statistics on Australian fructose consumption are harder to come across. We don't have an equivalent of the US Department of Agriculture fastidiously compiling 'food disappearance data'. But from the data we do have, our consumption is significantly lower than in the United States. In 1999, every person in Australia ate just under 38kg of sugar. This seems mostly to be related to the fact that we drink only half as much carbonated soft drink as our American friends. But we are catching up fast. Soft-drink consumption increased by 30 per cent in the '90s alone. We prefer to support our cane farmers rather than our corn farmers, so very little HFCS is used in Australia.

Add the fructose from the sugar (19kg) to the 3.5kg we were getting from juices, and it means Australians were consuming about 22.5kg of fructose by the turn of the twenty-first century. It's not as bad as the 33kg the Americans were guzzling, but it's still an awful lot more than the less than zero kilos of added fructose we were eating 130 years before that. A lot of the people conducting experiments on rats had been criticised for giving the animals unrealistically high doses of fructose. 'Of course the rat would die. Look how much fructose you gave it,' would be the cry. 'No person actually eats that much fructose.' These figures tell a different story. Every man, woman and child in the United States (and Australia) is eating that much fructose and more. The USDA rats were actually on lower fructose diets than most of the people feeding them.

This was getting really scary. If we were all really eating that much fructose, and fructose really had the effects on us that the medical research suggested, we were in real trouble. Given that the average American adult was eating 33kg of fructose every year, and that since fructose subverts our appetite control and creates fat immediately, 33kg would be directly converted to almost 15kg of body fat every year, it was a significant miracle that everybody in the country wasn't clinically obese already. All the gyms, fitness crazes and diets were working to keep the inflation at a lower rate, but 'pushing water uphill with a rake' was a phrase that sprang to mind when they were viewed in the context of the fructose tidal wave. And while no-one was having to install larger seats in our airplanes to accommodate most Australians, the data suggested we were heading in that direction.

8. PORRIDGE IN THE ARTERIES

I was clinically obese when I started trying to understand the obscure world of medical research. I wanted to find out why I was fat and how I could reverse the process. Through many years of trial and error I had found out the hard way that nothing any diet guru said was ever likely to make any difference. My research had spurred me on to discover what William Banting had found 150 years before me – low-carbohydrate diets (like Atkins) were different. They worked, but were impossible to stick to in the long term unless I was prepared to transplant myself to a society that just ate meat (like the Alaskan Inuit before the western world showed them a 'better way'). But the research had revealed a lot more to me than why I was fat. A lot of those rat experiments were telling me that being fat was the least of my worries. Sure, fructose was making me fat, but these rats were suffering far worse fates than being giggled at by the other rats at the gym. They were dying of truly horrible diseases. Diseases that sounded like those that I had been reading about more and more in the newspaper. Things like heart disease, diabetes, stroke, liver cancer, pancreatic cancer and breast cancer.

I decided to do some digging on what research had been done on the association between some of these diseases and fructose consumption. The obvious place to start was obesity. It's the unequivocal sign that something is going wrong with our body. There is a lot of talk about the obesity epidemic in the media today, but rather than rely on the hype, I wanted to sort out exactly how fat we were all getting and how fast.

Researchers measure the extent to which we are overweight using a standard measure called the body mass index, or BMI. Our BMI is a number calculated from our weight in kilograms divided by the square of our height in centimetres.

The BMI formula was invented in about 1835 by Belgian mathematician and astronomer Lambert Quetelet. Quetelet was also responsible for starting Florence Nightingale on her one-woman crusade that changed the way sick people are cared for. He felt very strongly that probability should be applied to all sciences where there was an element of observation. Since absolute certainty was impossible when looking at large numbers of stars, rocks, animals or people, being able to apply probabilities rather than precise measurements would be handy. His theory was that people's measurements varied only so much. If you line up 100 people you would be extremely unlikely to come across anyone who was 10 metres tall. The height of a person varied within a range of limits that could be measured by looking at a sample of the population. Once he had the sample numbers he could apply his new probability theory to give an estimate of how many people in the whole population were what height. The same process could be applied to other measurements, such as weight.

In 1825, Quetelet started publishing papers on what he called social statistics: studies on crime rates, birth, death and marriage rates, and human physical appearance. He was the first to collect large amounts of data on these subjects and apply statistical methods to them. To ensure he had a standard basis for comparison for the data he was collecting about human height and weight, he devised the Quetelet index and published it in 1835 in what was the first statistical population study of human appearance. The index allowed Quetelet to compare directly the weight of two people of different heights and genders. The Quetelet index is now called the body mass index, or BMI.

BMI provides a reliable indicator of the amount of body fat for most people. An adult is considered overweight when their BMI lies in the range 25 to 29.9, and obese when it is 30 or more.

I am 1.8m (5 feet 11 inches) tall. When I started looking for answers, I weighed in at a hefty 120kg. According to the BMI graph (over the page), I was well into the obese zone. As I write this, I am 80kg, which means that I have just slipped into the top of the normal zone. The BMI is not a definitive tool that should be applied strictly. It was developed as a way of statistically comparing large populations of individuals, not as a method for individual diagnosis. There could be all manner of reasons why a particular person is outside a given band in the BMI chart but not actually over- or underweight. Body composition, for example the amount of muscle versus fat, will affect the measure. Muscle is denser than fat so elite athletes will record higher BMI numbers than the rest of us. But being mistaken for an elite athlete has never been one of my problems.

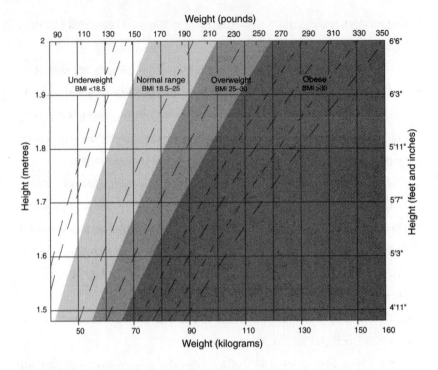

Figure 8.1: The BMI chart – simply locate the point where your height crosses with your weight to see which range your BMI lies in.

Race can also make a difference. Caucasians and people of African descent can rely on the BMI as being fairly accurate, but the World Health Organization has recently recommended that for people with a South-East Asian body type, the cut-off between healthy and overweight should be lowered from 25 to 23. That being said, the BMI is a fairly reliable indicator of population trends and a very solid indicator of how we measure up as a population. It also provides a relatively accurate way of comparing the population over time because even if the BMI wasn't explicitly calculated when the data was collected, most health surveys do record weight and height statistics, which allows BMIs to be calculated long after the research has been published and the participants have gone home (although you have to watch out for the studies where these were self-reported rather than measured – we are all taller and thinner when we fill in survey forms).

BMI ranges are based on adult sizings. BMI figures are different for children and are dependent on their age. As a general rule of thumb, a two-year-old child is regarded as obese when their BMI hits 18 (rather than 30 for an adult). And that threshold increases gradually until an 18-year-old has the same limit as an adult.

If you look at BMI calculations over time you quickly realise that the obesity epidemic is very real and is a very recent phenomenon. The United States has been keeping comprehensive health data on their population for longer than most other nations, so a lot of the examples I use are based on their data. As the rest of the world started to catch up, we got better at keeping statistics, so where I can, I have supplemented the US data with more modern examples from the rest of the world.

In 1910, just over one in five US adults was overweight and fewer than one in five of those people was obese (one in 25 for the whole population). Less than a century later, two out of every three US adults are overweight and half of those people are now obese (one-third of the whole population). In less than 100 years, the chances of a given US adult being overweight have gone from very unlikely to highly probable, and the trend is accelerating. It took half a century to double the percentage of overweight people in the US population. Forty years later, it had almost doubled again. If the obesity epidemic continues at its current pace, four out of five of the US Generation X (born 1966–1975) will be obese (not just overweight – obese) by age 70, in around 2036. By then, a person with a normal BMI will be as rare as an eight-leaf clover.

Don't laugh too loud at the Americans. In Australia, our statistics are just as shocking. By the year 2000, just over 60 per cent of the Australian adult population was overweight or obese. In 2000, one

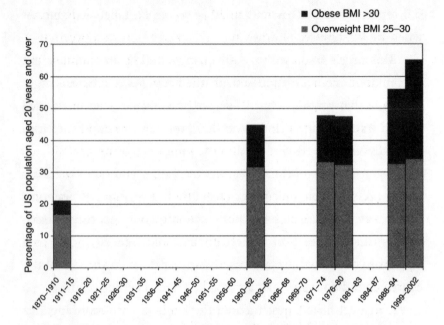

Figure 8.2: The percentage of overweight and obese adults in the United States, as recorded in intermittent studies. In the space of less than a century, the number of overweight people has tripled, and the number of them that are obese is seven times as high.

in five adults in Australia was clinically obese. Just two decades earlier, only one in 14 Australian adults was obese. We aren't yet at the US benchmark of one in three, but we are eating hard to get there.

We are now statistically more likely to be overweight than not. According to the World Health Organization, a billion of the world's 6 billion people are now considered overweight and 30 per cent of those people are obese. The vast majority are concentrated in the United States and Europe, but the rest of the world is catching up fast. In Europe it's almost one in two – 200 million – adults that is measurably overweight. Even in European countries where obesity is less prevalent, the percentage has increased steadily in recent times. In France, with a population of just over 60 million, 5.9 million people are obese today, whereas the figure just 10 years ago was only

3.6 million. In China, more than 20 per cent of the people in certain cities (the westernised ones) are now classified as seriously overweight.

This acceleration in weight gain is not limited to adults. The percentage of young people in the United States who are overweight has more than tripled since 1980. Among children and teens aged six to 19 years, 16 per cent (over 9 million young people) are considered overweight. There are about 14 million overweight pre-teen children in the European Union and at least 3 million of them are obese, according to a recent study by the International Task Force on Obesity. In Portugal, for example, more than 30 per cent of nine- to 16-year-olds are obese, three times more than a decade ago. Approximately 5 to 7 per cent of Australian children are currently estimated to be obese.

Like you, I had heard all these numbers (or something like them) before. Barely a news bulletin goes by without some politician bleating about how fat we are all getting or some nutritional genius telling us about the next great discovery that will stop us getting fat. You stop hearing the detail and the fact that we are all getting fatter becomes background noise. But once I understood where the fat was coming from – fructose – I started paying attention. We were getting fatter, a lot fatter – and very, very quickly. If obesity was a disease like bird flu, we'd be bunkered down with a shotgun and three years' supply of baked beans in the garage. But nobody actually dies from obesity itself. You never hear of anyone being pronounced dead from being fat. No, people die from other diseases that may or may not be related to being fat, like cardiovascular disease (heart attack and stroke), kidney failure or various cancers. Obesity is a symptom, not a disease.

Some diseases are directly related to increased body mass, such as osteoarthritis and fractures (due to increased pressure on joints and bones), hernia and sleep apnoea (the treatment for which is becoming a huge industry), but these are relatively insignificant when compared with the mass murderers of modern society. The biggest killer in Australia today is cardiovascular disease (CVD). It is almost completely attributable to blocked arteries, or, more medically, atherosclerosis (from the Greek *athera*, meaning porridge – because that's what it looks like – and *skleros*, meaning hard, leading to the rather descriptive 'arterial hardness caused by porridge'. Sounds better in Greek, doesn't it?). These blockages are formed from the exact fatty acids created in overabundance by the consumption of fructose. The percentage of the population suffering from these diseases has risen in direct parallel (with a 55-year time lag) with the acceleration in fructose consumption.

In Australia, 48,000 people will die from a CVD this year, over 30 times as many as will die in a car accident and over 300 times as many as will die from AIDS. In the United States, around 650 000 people will die from a CVD this year. One and a half million Australians are estimated to be living with a disability associated with a CVD. The name of the particular CVD that threatens or takes your life depends largely on which major organ is nearby the 'porridge' blocking your artery. The organ system needing treatment also determines which type of specialist operates on you (if you make it to the hospital).

One CVD alone, ischaemic heart disease (IHD), is responsible for 63 per cent of the CVD deaths in Australia today. IHD is also often referred to as coronary heart disease, or CHD. IHD is a reduced blood supply to the heart, usually caused by atherosclerosis blocking the coronary arteries that supply the heart. It usually takes about 50 to 60 years to accumulate a life-threatening blockage, which is why very few people under the age of 40 suffer heart attacks. A symptom of IHD is increased blood pressure, or hypertension. One of the known effects of insulin is that it causes the arteries to dilate in healthy people, which normally causes a lowering of blood pressure. When a person's blood is filled with excess fatty acids, however, they become insulin resistant, resulting in arteries not dilating in response to insulin. Many researchers now believe that this failure to dilate may be the cause of a significant percentage of hypertension cases. Another symptom is angina, caused by the heart having to cope with a reduced blood supply. Angina is a warning sign that the artery is dangerously blocked. Enough blood can get through the narrow opening for normal daily needs, but when more blood is needed in a hurry (usually because of exercise or stress) and not enough can get through, the temporary chest pains called angina ensue.

A more definitive symptom is myocardial infarction (MI). MI is the classic sudden-death heart attack we see all the time on TV – clutching the chest, our hero falls to the street and is pronounced dead by the not-quite-on-time ambulance crew. This year, one quarter of all Australians with heart disease will experience their first-ever symptom (a fatal MI) within the hour before they die. An MI is generally caused by the porridge (which has a hard skin) rupturing and squirting fatty acids into the blood at the site of the rupture. This usually induces a blood clot that either blocks the artery totally or causes the heart muscle to die. Either way, the end result is a heart attack.

It is very difficult to obtain accurate historical data on the rates of heart attack, mostly because MI wasn't even recognised as a medical problem until 1912 (due to its rarity – but more on that shortly). And what caused it wasn't nailed down with any certainty until the 1920s. In some very rare instances, though, researchers have been very lucky. When accurate records are kept about people's births and deaths, it is possible to construct a complete cradle-to-grave analysis of a whole set of lives lived. When the data is old enough, researchers can proceed with some certainty about causes of death because everybody they are studying is now dead. One such study was completed in the late '90s by Australian researchers seeking to determine if there was a relationship between low birth weights and death by heart disease. They found there wasn't, but in the process they used the excellent death registry created by William Henry Archer to compile an extensive database of causes of death in the early Australian colonies.

When William Henry Archer, a statistician by training, was demoted from his position of managing actuary at the Catholic, Law and General Life Assurance Company of London in 1852, he decided to throw in the job and move his family to the new colony at Port Phillip Bay, Australia. His rare statistical training stood him in good stead with the governor and, in 1853, he was appointed to the newly created position of Registrar of Births, Deaths and Marriages for Her Majesty's Colony of Victoria. Archer is credited with creating one of the most detailed and accurate databases of births, deaths and marriages in the world.

Archer's database was used by the researchers in conjunction with the records of what is now the Royal Women's Hospital in Melbourne to create a complete dataset for the lives of people born at that hospital between 1857 and 1900 who survived beyond the age of 40 (almost 3000 people).

The age-adjusted dataset reveals that prior to 1930 less than 2 per cent of people had died from symptoms that today would be diagnosed as an IHD-induced MI (heart attack). From 1930 to 1949 about four times as many (8 per cent) died from the condition.

From 1950 to 1959, the figure jumped to 27 per cent, more than 10 times as much as it had been just two decades earlier. And 55 years after the introduction of sugar use in commercial quantities, almost 30 per cent of deaths were attributable to heart attacks caused by the blockage of the arteries with fats. Exactly the same fats that we now know are produced as a direct result of the consumption of fructose.

There are many problems with relying too much on a study done in this way with such a comparatively small and old dataset, but the results do match up with similar work done in the United States. The US studies suggest that MI was almost nonexistent as a cause of death in 1900 and caused no more than 3000 deaths per year by 1930. Dr Paul Dudley White, who introduced the electrocardiograph machine to America, said during a 1956 American Heart Association televised fund-raiser: 'I began my practice as a cardiologist in 1921 and I never saw an MI patient until 1928.' By 1960, there were at least half a million MI deaths per year in the United States.

The other major variant of CVD that kills thousands of people every year is stroke (cerebral infarction). A stroke is a disruption of the blood supply to the brain. Just like atherosclerosis of the arteries leading to the heart, when the arteries leading to the brain fill with porridge, blood supply is reduced. Sometimes the atherosclerosis ruptures and produces a clot that completely blocks blood supply to part of the brain. Brain cells can survive about four minutes without the oxygen that the blood supply brings. After that, brain-cell death near the site of the blockage begins. Depending on how long treatment is in coming or whether the blood supply is completely blocked, stroke is more survivable than MI. Only one in three stroke sufferers dies as a direct result of the stroke (compared with 90 per cent of MI sufferers). However, they do not generally escape without some brain damage as a result; only 10 per cent return to normal. About 15 per cent of all hospital beds and one-quarter of all nursing-home beds are filled with survivors of stroke at any given time. Unlike the heart, there are many entry points for blood supply to the brain, and strokes tend to have local effects that then slowly spread. Around 12 000 Australians will die this year from strokes. Just as with heart attacks, not all strokes are caused by atherosclerosis, but they account for the majority by far – more than 80 per cent.

Atherosclerosis is obviously not confined to arteries that supply the brain and the heart. It can and does occur anywhere in the body (especially the legs), but a blockage in most other locations, while serious, is not normally as deadly, with 'only' 2500 Australians expected to die in 2008 as a result of those types of blockages. That's still more than the national road toll, but it pales into insignificance against the 37 000 dying from heart attack and stroke.

Modern statistics reveal that the number of people dying from a CVD peaked in about 1968 – at almost 65 per cent of the total number of deaths that year – and has been declining since then to the current 30 per cent. The decline is uniform across all age groups, both sexes and in all first-world countries. Followers of the anti-fat message of Dr Ancel Keys have been quick to claim the credit for the decline. A closer look at the data reveals that the primary cause is just plain old-fashioned economics rather than a reduction in the amount of fat we eat. Don't get me wrong, there is nothing wrong with eating less fat (and in doing so, you will definitely reduce the amount of circulating fatty acids in your system), it's just that your body is already capable of controlling how much fat you eat and it is relatively unimportant as a source of fatty acids if you also continue to eat fructose.

The decline in deaths is actually attributable to a lot of money and the better medicine that it buys. In 1924, six American doctors (one of them being Dr Paul Dudley White – the chap who was not to see an MI until 1928) formed the American Heart Association (AHA), a small scientific society aimed at promoting public interest in heart disease. With MI causing less than 10 per cent of deaths at the time, the public was unbelievably ignorant about the disease, to paraphrase Dr White. The AHA remained relatively obscure for 25 years, relying on dues from its (mostly medical) members. Its annual budget never exceeded $50 000 during that time. In 1948, that all changed very suddenly when the AHA successfully managed to lobby the US government to establish the National Heart Institute (NHI). A significant factor in its success was the fact that, by then, one in three American deaths was caused by a CVD. CVDs were clearly at epidemic proportions and urgent action was needed. At the same time, the AHA transformed itself into a voluntary health agency and became a major recipient of NHI-controlled funds to develop expertise in CVD research. The AHA had transformed itself from an obscure scientific society to a major distributor of research grants for heart disease research, all courtesy of an epidemic that was clearly spiralling out of control. Today the AHA employs 2500 full-time staff and 4.5 million volunteers, and boasts a membership of over 30 000. It is the second-largest not-for-profit health agency in the world. The AHA raises over $400 million every year and spends over $100 million a year funding or supplementing government funding for medical research on heart disease, as well as its own internal research and education programs.

In 1968, two decades after the NHI was established and the AHA transformed, things were not going so well. By then, two out of every three American deaths were caused by a CVD and the story was similar in most of the developed world. CVDs were obviously an extreme priority for government and private health spending alike. The AHA and the NHI had spent 20 years pouring money into research and seriously multiplying the number of cardiologists, and eventually cardiac surgeons, by creating vast numbers of academic stipends to encourage the teaching of cardiology. The only result by then was a doubling in the number of deaths due to CVD, but the spending was about to pay off. Since 1968, the number of deaths due to CVD has more than halved. This number of deaths is still significant, but it means we have now put ourselves back in the position we were in when the AHA and the NHI started out – 'only' one in three deaths are due to a CVD.

In 1964, the age of intervention in the treatment of arterial disease dawned with the first successful use of a balloon-tipped catheter to treat atherosclerosis in a leg artery. Before this, the primary treatment for CVD was to be put into a hospital bed until you died (rather like type I diabetes before the discovery of insulin). The new catheter treatment involved inserting a thin tube into the artery and threading it to the point of the blockage. The balloon was then inflated against the blocked area to create a wider passage for blood flow. It wasn't tried on a heart artery until 1977, but it was so successful that less than a decade later 300 000 such operations were being performed every year in the United States. The first balloon catheter operation was performed in Australia in 1980. That year, 11 in total were performed. By 1986, technology had developed to the point where the first stent was implanted: a metal or synthetic mesh cylinder inserted after the balloon catheter has widened the artery, to prevent it from narrowing again. By the turn of the century, 20 000 Australian balloon catheter operations were being performed every year.

In 1967, Rene Favalaro, an Argentine cardiac surgeon working at the Cleveland Clinic, in Ohio, was pioneering the other significant advance in heart disease treatment, a surgical technique whereby a blockage was bypassed altogether using a grafted artery (usually) from the patient's leg. By 1980, almost 4000 Australian bypass operations were being performed annually. And by the turn of the century, that number had increased almost fivefold to nearly 18 000 per year. In 2007, around 500 000 bypass surgeries were performed in the United States.

The drug companies were not going to miss out on the biggest public health spending bonanza in history. They started research immediately and by the late '80s were able to release a raft of new drugs targeting cholesterol and blood pressure. Consumption of many of these drugs increased eightfold in the decade that followed and continues to climb rapidly.

The development of the surgical techniques and drugs has been a worldwide phenomenon, with all first-world nations implementing these major interventionist techniques shortly after their first successful trials.

It is important to note that prevalence (the number of people with a disease in the population) of CVDs has not decreased. In Australia, it continues to increase at a rate of about 2 per cent per annum, about twice the rate of population growth. And blood cholesterol levels remain just as high as they were in 1980, when such things first started being measured; about 50 per cent of the population continues to have high blood cholesterol. We haven't cured anything; we are just better at making sure fewer people die from it. The medical profession has shown us the difference between an untreated CVD and a treated CVD. If it's not treated, it accounts for two in every three deaths. If vast amounts of money are thrown at the problem, we can get that down to one in every three deaths. I suspect we have reached the limits of technology to solve the problem and we are about to face another acceleration in the death rates, because nothing has been done about the major underlying cause.

When you break the figures down by gender, women seem to have an advantage. Pre-menopausal women are half as likely as men to suffer from a CVD. After menopause they catch up, and if they (and the men) lived to be 90, they would both have the same chance of death due to a CVD. This suggests to me that there is something protective about being a woman in so far as the effect that fructose has on the production of circulating fatty acids. Many of the rat researchers noticed the same thing. Male rats fared much worse in the fructose feeding than female rats of breeding age. Females beyond breeding age lost their protection and suffered just as much as their male counterparts.

Up to the age of 35, there are fewer overweight women than men and they are less likely to suffer a CVD when they are

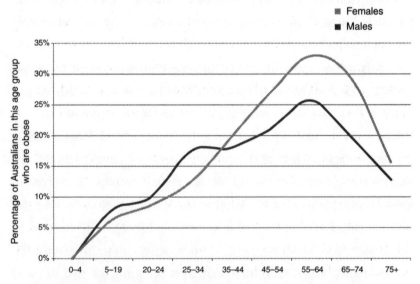

Figure 8.3: 2005 Australian figures for the percentage of women and men in each age category who are obese – women have an advantage before menopause, but then well and truly make up for it afterwards. The stats drop off after 65 because the really obese people are dying by then.

pre-menopausal. But 40 years later, they are in just as much trouble as the men. It appears that there is something about the interaction of female reproductive hormones and fructose metabolism that favours immediate body-fat creation rather than increased circulating cholesterol levels. Researchers at the Mayo Clinic Endocrine Research Unit in Rochester, Minnesota, have published the results of limited trials they performed in 1995, which showed that oestrogen helps fat cells vacuum fatty acids out of the bloodstream. This means that, if you happen to have oestrogen in your blood (bad luck, gentlemen), the fatty acids created by fructose will be more efficiently turned into body fat rather than hanging around in the bloodstream and making bowls of porridge in the arteries. While this may be very bad news for women seeking to fit into this year's bikini, it is probably good news for their chances of being killed by a CVD (or any of the other diseases we are about to discuss).

More recent research, conducted in 2002 by the Division of Geriatric Medicine at the University of Colorado, found that oestrogen also seemed to make insulin work more efficiently in clearing the blood of glucose. To prove this they injected post-menopausal women with oestrogen and measured the before and after differences in how efficiently the insulin did its work. This interaction between fructose (or at least the fatty acids it produces) and female reproductive hormones has also been put forward by some researchers as a possible reason for the recent rapid decline in the age of female sexual maturity, with girls hitting puberty much younger than their mothers and grandmothers did. It is very early days for research in this area, and certainly too early to make any definitive conclusions, but I am watching it with interest.

CVDs are not a high-publicity set of diseases. Even though they kill huge numbers of people, the victims are mostly elderly. In the last five decades or so, we have become inured to the concept of people dying of heart attacks or eventually from strokes. After all, we've all got to go somehow and that's how most people seem to die. Advances in medical treatment have meant that there is no obvious impact of the escalation of these diseases (yet), such as there suddenly being no way to live past 60. And it doesn't affect the lifestyles of the young and newsworthy. You can have a CVD your whole life and the first you will be aware of it is when you suffer the first fatal symptom. The build-up of arterial porridge is a slow-accumulation disease with a very decisive outcome, but often no degradation of lifestyle before that point.

9. MORE KILLERS

Cardiovascular diseases are not the only new diseases our love affair with fructose has created. Type II diabetes was rarer than CVDs in 1900 and, compared with CVDs, still doesn't kill a large number of people today. In 2008, 3500 Australians were expected to die because of diabetes (twice as many as would be killed on our roads) and another 8500 from CVDs where diabetes has been a contributing factor. But there are two things about diabetes that make it much more newsworthy than CVDs. It affects younger people and, while it doesn't necessarily kill them, it significantly affects their lifestyle. Unlike CVDs, as long as it is treated, diabetes takes a long time to kill the patient. A diabetic will usually only die after a lifetime of altered or truncated living, complicated by some non-fatal but very nasty side effects.

Around one in 350 people in Australia suffers from type I diabetes, and that number (as a percentage of the population) has not changed significantly over time. Whatever is wrongly identifying the islets of Langerhans as viruses and destroying them in type I diabetics has not changed significantly in the century or so that statistics on such things have been kept. Type II diabetes is a different beast altogether. The outcome is the same, but the cause is very well documented and in many cases preventable. The number of people with type II diabetes is accelerating rapidly. Type II diabetes was once called late-onset diabetes because it normally only affected old people. But as the number of fat people in the population has increased and the population of fat people has become younger, it is now becoming common in people in their 20s and increasingly occurring in teenagers and even children.

The disease is caused by the body becoming immune to the effects of insulin. Insulin is still being manufactured (often in huge quantities) but the body becomes resistant to it, requiring more and more insulin to remove the amount of glucose building up in the blood. Studies on rats, hamsters and dogs, as well as some limited human trials conducted during the last 30 years, have proved that fructose consumption results in insulin resistance even when maintained for only short periods of time. The rapid increase in circulating fat caused by the fructose metabolism inhibits insulin's ability to instruct cells that require energy to take the glucose out of the bloodstream. Eventually, either the body cannot manufacture enough insulin to remove the glucose, or the islets of Langerhans wear out from overuse and their capacity to produce insulin significantly reduces. The result is the same as for type I diabetes: the body starves in a sea of food.

Insulin resistance is a preliminary phase of type II diabetes. When a person is insulin resistant, their blood-sugar levels remain high for longer than would be expected after eating a meal. This is a sign that the body is struggling to dispose of the glucose. The body has become resistant to the effects of insulin. If insulin resistance is left untreated, it eventually develops into full-blown diabetes, where no matter how much insulin is produced, the blood-sugar levels remain permanently too high.

The prevalence of type II diabetes is now increasing so rapidly that the Centers for Disease Control and Prevention and the World Health Organization characterise it as an epidemic. The International Diabetes Federation estimated that in 2003 about 194 million people worldwide, or 5.1 per cent of the adult population, had diabetes, and that this will almost double to 333 million by 2025. The number of people with confirmed insulin resistance was estimated at 314 million in 2003 and is expected to increase to 472 million by 2025. In less than two decades, almost 1 billion people worldwide will be affected by a potentially life-threatening disease that was virtually unheard of less than 30 years ago. What's worse is that these figures are likely to be underestimates (they have already been revised upwards by

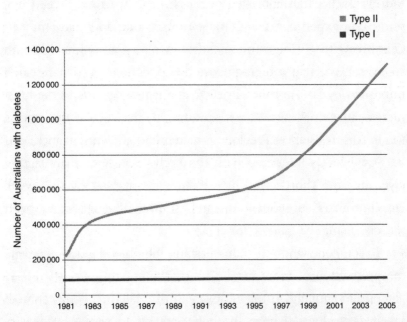

Figure 9.1: The number of Australians with type II diabetes has exploded in the last 25 years. The disease is now at epidemic proportions.

11 per cent since the predictions were first made in 2001). In some cultures, the future is already here. Polynesians, Aboriginal Australians and Native Americans seem particularly susceptible to the effects of prolonged insulin resistance and prevalence rates are soaring. With type II diabetes now affecting up to half of some populations of these indigenous peoples, they are now five times as likely to die from diabetes as Caucasians. In New Zealand, for example, one in five Maori deaths is as a direct result of diabetes, compared with one in 20 in the Caucasian population.

One of the things the USDA's Sheldon Reiser and his team noticed during their experiments in feeding rats too much fructose during the late '70s was that the rats on 27 per cent fructose diets developed insulin resistance after a relatively short time (two to four weeks). The results were confirmed in 1989 by Dr AW Thorburn and his colleagues at the St Vincent's Institute in Sydney, using a four-week diet that consisted of 35 per cent fructose. Since then, numerous experiments with rats, rabbits and dogs have proved definitively that a high-fructose diet increases an animal's insulin resistance, whereas a high-glucose diet does not. Further research published by Dr Thorburn in 2002 confirmed that it was the huge increase in circulating fatty acids induced by the fructose that caused the insulin resistance. Previous research had shown that increased fatty-acid levels interfered with the body's ability to manufacture glycogen (the short-term glucose store maintained by the liver). Dr Thorburn's subsequent research showed that it also stopped muscles using the glucose for energy.

In someone who is insulin resistant, high blood glucose triggers the production of more insulin in an attempt to lower the blood glucose. Eventually, in the early stages of type II diabetes, enough insulin is produced to break through the resistance caused by the fatty acids and lower the glucose levels. If this pattern of overproduction is maintained for years on end, eventually either the body cannot make enough insulin to lower the blood glucose levels or the islets of Langerhans become permanently damaged. There are some lines of modern research that suggest that the presence of fatty acids may itself directly damage the islets, but at this stage that is speculation. From our perspective, it doesn't matter whether the effect is direct or indirect: the result is the same. It is still not clear exactly how the fatty acids interfere with the action of insulin, but it is beyond doubt that the massive increase in fatty acid production, induced by eating fructose, does cause insulin resistance and eventually leads to type II diabetes. It seems the results are now in from our own little fructose-feeding experiment. If you feed millions of humans massive quantities of fructose for the first 20 to 30 years of their lives, you can create a type II diabetes epidemic.

Type II diabetes affects men much more than it does pre-menopausal women. The oestrogen research described in the previous chapter probably goes a long way to explaining why. Oestrogen helps clear the fatty acids that cause insulin resistance, and it also appears that it helps insulin do its work even more directly by accelerating the absorption of glucose. If you have oestrogen in your veins, it will take a lot more fructose to give you type II diabetes than if you don't.

Accumulation of fat in the arteries starts happening from the very first extra gram of fructose (or fat) consumed. Fifty to 60 years of continuous fructose feeding leads to a high likelihood of a heart attack or stroke. The rapid increase in fructose consumption we have all been part of in the last 30 years has probably accelerated that process, meaning that heart attacks and strokes may start to occur in younger and younger people. Type II diabetes is different. It appears that we can tolerate a certain level of fat in the blood caused by fructose and not develop the disease – we can overproduce insulin at a certain level without shutting down the islets of Langerhans. Thirty years after fructose consumption began increasing due to the introduction of soft drinks to our diet in the early '50s, Type II diabetes started a mirror-image climb. If the type II diabetes curve is in fact a mirror of the fructose curve, 30 years delayed, there is much worse news to come on the diabetes front.

Over the last 30 years alone, type II diabetes has changed from being seen as a relatively mild and rare ailment associated with ageing and the elderly to one of the major contemporary causes of premature death in most countries. In virtually every developed society, type II diabetes is the leading cause of blindness, kidney failure and lower limb amputation (3000 diabetes-related amputations were expected to be performed in Australia in 2008) and is a significant risk factor for death from heart disease. Worldwide, there is a death due to type II diabetes every 10 seconds, and an amputation every 30 seconds. And there are predictions that the disease will single-handedly wipe out whole races of indigenous peoples in the Pacific within 100 years.

Diabetes is not as suddenly fatal as CVDs. It generally debilitates over an extended period before it kills. Just as with type I diabetes, too much sugar in the blood, over a decade or so, causes permanent damage to the fine blood vessels in the kidneys, eyes, arms and legs, often resulting in blindness, kidney damage and amputations. People with diabetes tend to live with a significantly reduced and eroding quality of life. Unlike with CVDs, the good news is that, if caught early, insulin resistance and even type II diabetes can be reversed before permanent damage is done. Animal experiments have shown that very shortly after fructose feeding ceases, the fatty acids in the blood reduce and insulin resistance subsides. If insulin overproduction (because of resistance) remains untreated for prolonged periods, eventually permanent damage is done to the islets of Langerhans and this cannot be reversed. When this occurs, the person has effectively turned themselves into a type I diabetic and can no longer produce any, or sufficient, insulin for their needs.

Fatal diabetes-induced kidney failure occurs in 15 per cent of sufferers, and it seems there's even worse news for males with excess long-term fructose consumption. Dr Reiser's rat studies noted enlarged testes, enlarged male breasts, decreased libido, impotence and decreased sperm production among the plethora of rather nasty outcomes for his furry male subjects. These results have been confirmed recently by the advent of yet another significant new chronic disease related to fructose consumption. Besides type II diabetes, insulin resistance also results in the development of non-alcoholic fatty liver disease (NAFLD). NAFLD is an accumulation of fatty acids in liver cells that causes enlargement of the organ. In extreme cases it can cause the cells to burst; the scar tissue that forms around the burst cells is called cirrhosis. If enough of the liver's normal mass is replaced by scar tissue, cirrhosis is ultimately fatal (over 35000 Americans and 1500 Australians died of cirrhosis in 2007, of which it is estimated 18 per cent are thought to be due to NAFLD).

Studies are now beginning to confirm Dr Reiser's observations, that a significant percentage of males with fructose-induced cirrhosis of the liver will experience testicular atrophy (the testes diminish in size and cease to function), impotence (no wonder there's such a demand for pills that assist in this department) and enlarged male breasts. Research conducted collaboratively in 2007 by teams in Italy and Britain have confirmed that 70 per cent of type II diabetes patients will suffer from NAFLD and that patients with a CVD are very likely to have the disease even when they don't exhibit any of the other commonly accepted risk factors for CVD (eating lots of fat, smoking, being overweight, etc.). Because of the relative newness of type II diabetes and insulin resistance as major diseases, there has been very little study of NAFLD, but early work suggests that it is becoming alarmingly common, particularly in children. It is estimated that up to 24 per cent of the US population now suffers from NAFLD.

The group of diseases and symptoms associated with heart attacks, stroke, type II diabetes and NAFLD are called metabolic syndrome. It is easy to see how fructose consumption can result in this syndrome – all of the conditions that fall under its umbrella relate directly to a single source: increased circulating fatty acids. And we know that fructose is converted into fatty acids.

But there is another set of major killers that some researchers believe are also connected to fructose, or at least to the fatty acids they produce. The set of diseases that kills just about everybody that CVDs and diabetes don't get are the cancers.

Dr Yudkin noticed that there was a high correlation between obesity and the likelihood that a person would end up suffering from some types of cancer. He cautioned strongly against drawing too many conclusions from statistics (obviously a believer in the line 'lies, damned lies and statistics') but he felt it was worth noting that there were strong correlations between obesity and colorectal, breast, kidney and prostate cancers.

Cancer is a large and diverse group of diseases potentially affecting every part of the human body. A cancer occurs when the mechanism that controls cell reproduction becomes defective and cells multiply out of control. When this happens, the cancerous cells can invade and damage the tissue around them. Cancer is never good, but it can be very, very bad if it occurs in or near a vital organ.

Cancers are named for the systems that they affect. There are over 200 types of cancer, but just five of them account for almost 90 per cent of all new cases. They are (in order of mortality rate): lung cancer, melanoma, colorectal (bowel) cancer, breast cancer and prostate cancer. We have a very solid idea about what causes two of those. Too much sunshine causes melanoma. And too much smoking causes lung cancer. The other three are cancers that Dr Yudkin noticed correlated with sugar intake.

Over 101 000 Australians were expected to be diagnosed with cancer in 2008 (excluding non-melanoma skin cancers, which account for a further 374 000 cases), and about 38 000 people will die from cancer. The biggest killer is lung cancer, but the rate of death per 100 000 people has declined significantly in the last two decades.

The next biggest killers are breast and colorectal cancers. They are the second and third most common cancers (respectively) worldwide, with two-thirds of all colorectal and breast cancers occurring in the more developed nations. There is a huge variation in rates of colorectal and breast cancer from country to country, but it is always the case that if one is high, then so is the other. The lowest rates are in Africa and Asia (except Japan) and the highest in Europe, North America and Australasia. Both cancers are definitively related to the western diet. Studies of people moving from less developed countries to the United States have shown that there is a rapid increase in risk for colorectal and breast cancer in those migrants, and the rates for second-generation migrants can be double that of first-generation migrants. Countries that have had a rapid westernisation

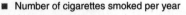
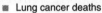
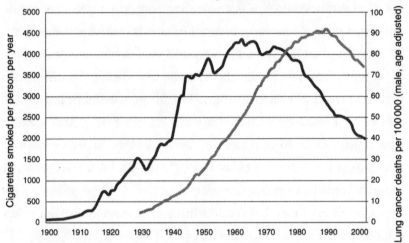

Figure 9.2: The number of cigarettes smoked per person per day in the United States compared with the number of lung cancer deaths per 100 000 men over the last century.

of their diet, such as Japan, have seen a rapid increase in the incidence of both cancers.

As soon as the diet link was noticed, the usual suspects were rolled out, with the Keys adherents declaring that increased fat consumption was obviously the cause. This was modified later to be increased meat consumption after correlations with fat proved inconclusive, and then later still to insufficient fruit and vegetable (fibre) consumption.

This last observation may not be too far from the mark. The mountain of money that found its way into CVD research in the '70s and '80s has recently had some side benefits for cancer research. A clear association has been established between insulin resistance and CVD as a result of the Insulin Resistance Atherosclerosis Study (funded by the successor to the National Heart Institute, the National Heart, Lung and Blood Institute) conducted in the United States in the early '90s. In-depth analysis in 2003 of the response to questionnaires from that study by researchers from the Department of Epidemiology (medical statistics) at the universities of South Carolina, Minnesota and Wake Forest confirmed the subsidiary conclusion from the original study, that fibre increases insulin sensitivity. This means that fibre has the same protective effect with regard to insulin use as oestrogen. Maybe Surgeon-Captain Cleave was on to something with his bags of bran after all? Both fibre and oestrogen appear to enhance the body's ability to use insulin to overcome the effect of circulating fatty acids and remove them and glucose from the bloodstream.

The observation that insulin resistance is related to increases in colorectal and breast cancers has been followed up with studies aimed at finding out why that is the case. A few of the studies are now starting to click together to form an overall theory.

In 1931, a German cell biologist called Otto Warburg picked up the Nobel Prize in Medicine for a little theory he had managed to prove in 1924. His theory concerned the way in which cancer cells derive energy from the bloodstream. He managed to prove that a cancerous cell uses glucose to produce energy directly and without oxygen. But it can only use glucose (rather than fat or protein) to do this. A normal cell requires the presence of oxygen to produce energy, but it can do so from glucose, fatty acids or proteins. Warburg theorised that this difference in cell biology was the cause of cancer and that all cancer was in fact due to defective cells that could not use oxygen to produce energy. More modern research based on studies of the genome have suggested that this in fact may be the cancerous cells adapting to a lack of oxygen inside a solid tumour, rather than a cause of cancer. Whether it is the cause or not, it is clear that cancerous cells consume more glucose than normal cells. Study after study in the '90s and early years of this century have shown that high blood-glucose levels are positively associated with cancer growth. In other words, the presence of high blood-glucose levels assists greatly in accelerating the growth of cancers. This is not to say that the glucose caused the cancer. There are likely to be as many causes as there are types of cancer. It is, however, clear that, whatever the cause, having a consistently high blood-glucose level accelerates the growth of cancerous cells.

High fatty-acid levels keep glucose levels high because the more fatty acids there are in the blood, the harder insulin has to work to remove them. Oestrogen and fibre are now known to be able to help insulin out by making insulin more efficient (we're still not sure how) and clearing the blood of glucose and fatty acids more quickly.

Pulling all of this together, we have a universal theory for what has been observed in a multitude of studies in the last three decades. Fructose increases circulating fatty acids, particularly LDL cholesterol. Increased fatty acids lead directly to heart disease and stroke. Increased fatty-acid levels also reduce the effectiveness of insulin in clearing the blood of glucose. Increased blood glucose leads to type II diabetes and feeds cancer. Oestrogen reduces (to a degree) the effects of fatty acids and allows insulin to work well despite their presence and to eliminate them from the bloodstream. This results in pre-menopausal women having lower incidences of heart disease, stroke, diabetes and cancer. Fibre has a similar effect to that of oestrogen (so there is hope for men after all) in rendering insulin more effective and therefore lowering the risk of all of those diseases. If you must eat fructose, then either have plenty of oestrogen on hand or eat a lot of fibre (hang on – fructose plus fibre . . . that sounds like whole fruit).

Because it has an obvious precursor (benign polyps in the bowel), colorectal cancer is almost completely avoidable as long as regular bowel checks are performed. This means the death rate for that cancer has decreased significantly in the last two decades. Prostate cancer is unfortunately incurable and there is very little evidence that any of the interventions tried so far significantly affect the rate of mortality. Comparing fructose consumption in the United States (because it has the best statistics) and prostate cancer reveals some alarming facts.

There has been a sharp downturn in mortality attributable to prostate cancer since 1990. And while the medical establishment would love to take the credit for it, study after study has failed to identify any treatment to which the trend can be attributed. Placing the trend on a graph as I have done below might help to provide an answer. The incidence of death from prostate cancer appears to be tracking (with a 60-year delay) the consumption of fructose in the US population. If that is in fact what is happening (and it certainly looks like it), then the current downturn in mortality relates

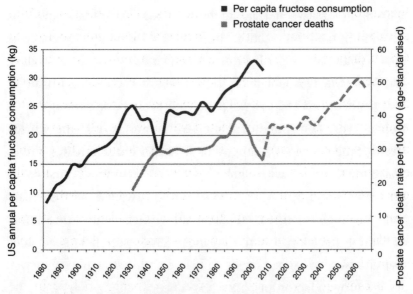

Figure 9.3: Prostate cancer rates appear to be tracking fructose consumption. The dashed line is a prediction calculated by me based on mortality continuing to track fructose consumption.

to the rationing of sugar that occurred during World War II, and the peak in the '90s was a consequence of the sugar binge between the depression and World War II. If the apparent trend continues, we should shortly expect to see a significant upswing in mortality rates as the baby boomers reach prostate cancer age.

It isn't a major problem in Australia yet, but a very new cancer on the hit list of killers is the one directly associated with the organ that produces insulin. Cancer of the pancreas strikes approximately five out of every 100 000 people every year in the United States and is one of the deadliest forms of cancer. With an estimated 32 180 Americans diagnosed with cancer of the pancreas in 2008, and with 31 800 deaths, mortality approaches 99 per cent. This adds up to pancreatic cancer having the number-one fatality rate of all cancers and shooting to number four on the hit list of cancer killers in the United States.

Two recently published large-scale studies have demonstrated a strong link between a diet high in fructose and the likelihood of developing pancreatic cancer. In 2002, Dr Dominique Michaud of the US National Cancer Institute, and Charles Fuchs of the Brigham and Women's Hospital and the Dana-Farber Cancer Institute in Boston, identified 180 cases of pancreatic cancer from among 88 802 women who were monitored for 18 years as part of the Nurses' Health Study. This is a longitudinal health characteristics survey that started in 1976 with a group of 121 700 registered nurses aged between 30 and 55. Women who were overweight and sedentary and had a high fructose intake were shown to be almost three times as likely to develop pancreatic cancer. The researchers speculated that glucose resistance may be to blame and that insulin may even act as a growth factor for pancreatic cancer.

A 2006 study published by the Karolinska Institute in Sweden has confirmed the results of the US Nurses' Health Study. The

Swedish study began in 1997 when scientists ran a dietary survey of almost 80 000 healthy people, who were subsequently monitored until June 2005. According to the cancer registry, 131 people from this group had developed cancer of the pancreas. The researchers have been able to demonstrate that the risk of developing pancreatic cancer is related to the amount of sugar in the diet. Most at risk were those who drank large quantities of soft drinks. The people who said that they drank such products twice a day or more were 90 per cent more likely to develop pancreatic cancer than those who never drank them. People who added sugar to food or drinks at least five times a day were at a 70 per cent greater risk than those who did not. People who ate fruit jams at least once a day also ran a higher risk – they developed the disease 50 per cent more often than those who never ate them.

The evidence linking sugar and cancer is starting to accumulate. Study after study associating sugar consumption and particular cancers is seeing the light of day. After decades looking for associations between fat or meat and cancers, researchers are producing consistent evidence that backs up Dr Yudkin's educated guess back in 1972 – sugar consumption is closely associated with cancer. I am taking that one step further and suggesting that the particular mechanism of that association is the fructose-induced fatty-acid accumulation that promotes a high-glucose environment. That environment is the perfect feeding ground for the growth of cancerous cells.

No chapter on the evil created by fructose would be complete without a quick look at the most obvious fructose-created condition of all. Every dentist will tell you not to eat sugar (and definitely not in liquid form) if you want to keep your teeth past the age of 35. The bacterial infection that causes tooth decay is the most common infection in humans. But nobody ever died of tooth decay. That and the fact that just about everybody has it has minimised its significance.

Researchers have known since the '60s that tooth decay is caused by just one (*Streptococcus mutans*, or SM) of the 200 to 300 species of bacteria that inhabit our mouths. In hundreds of very well-controlled studies, scientists were able to determine that feeding rats sucrose (table sugar) encouraged SM to produce decay, but feeding them pure glucose or fructose on their own did not. Microbiological studies conducted throughout the '70s and early '80s showed that SM needed both the glucose and the fructose present in sucrose. If both sugars were present, there was a perfect environment for SM to do its destructive work. Sucrose doesn't exist in any quantity in our natural environment (unless you are in the habit of sucking on sugarcane), so the discovery that sucrose was necessary for tooth decay went a long way towards explaining why dental cavities were not a significant medical problem before 1850. It also appears that SM prefers a constant supply of sucrose rather than big lumps at intervals. Unlike all the other conditions caused by sugar, tooth decay is not so much dependent on the quantity consumed, but rather the frequency of consumption. Constant snacking on sugar and sugar-laden drinks provides the perfect environment for SM, but a large amount of sugar at a mealtime doesn't help it much at all, especially if you are in the habit of cleaning your teeth after a meal. SM likes a sludge of sucrose to be present on the teeth at all times.

The costs associated with treating the symptoms of the activity of SM have grown exponentially in the past five decades (strangely coincident with the growth of the soft-drink industry). Governments, desperate to avoid the popular demand for them to pay the bill for a disease that affects everyone, have increasingly turned to the quick-fix solution of mass medication with fluoride.

We spend a lot of money fixing and treating (with varying degrees of success) the damage done by sugar. The Australian

Institute of Health and Welfare (a federal government department) has developed a sophisticated data-collection and analysis methodology for health-system cost measurement. According to AIHW numbers, in 2001, Australia spent $5.5 billion on CVDs, just short of $1 billion treating type II diabetes, another $2.9 billion on cancers, $3.4 billion on oral health (no wonder the government is keen on fluoride) and $1.5 billion on osteoarthritis. In addition to the $14.3 billion of annual direct costs, we spent at least that amount in lost productivity and other employment-related indirect costs to the economy. If you're like me, billions, trillions and gazillions are largely irrelevant without some basis for comparison. In the same year, we spent only $4 billion treating injuries and $3.7 billion on mental disorders (mostly Alzheimer's and dementia treatment in nursing homes). The amount directly spent on fructose- and sugar-induced disease in 2001 was just a little bit less than Australia spent on defence in 2005, even after paying for some less than cheap ongoing military deployments in Iraq, Timor and Afghanistan.

Drug companies love type II diabetes in particular. In Australia, 25 cents in every health dollar spent on diabetes goes directly into their pockets. In the United States in 2001, $3.5 billion was spent on drugs aimed at managing type II diabetes and it is easily the fastest-growing pharmaceutical market. The drugs do not cure the disease; they simply slow its progression (so the patient or, in Australia, the government has to buy the drugs over a longer period). The drugs generally either stimulate the pancreas to produce more insulin or increase insulin sensitivity. The real irony is that, of all the diseases I looked at, type II diabetes is the one that can be cured simply by not eating fructose (as long as it has not progressed to the point of destroying the islets of Langerhans).

Drug companies prefer to promote a slightly different message. Their message is that you can manage your insulin resistance by

stimulating the pancreas to produce more insulin. Much like fluori-
dation, it is an attack on the symptom rather than the cause.

Cholesterol-lowering drugs are in the same category. If you have
high cholesterol, try a little experiment. Stop eating fructose for two
weeks and see what happens to the fatty-acid levels in your blood.
You (and your GP) will be amazed. Doing this won't reverse your
accumulated atherosclerosis, but it will lower your LDL cholesterol
and blood triglyceride readings, and the reason is simple: you
will be removing the ingredient from your diet that most directly
produces them.

PART 2
WHAT CAN
YOU DO?

10. WHAT ABOUT EXERCISE?

You would have to look pretty hard to find a public-health message today that did not encourage you to exercise 'as part of a healthy lifestyle'. Exercise is now so tightly bound up with weight loss in the minds of governments, educators and the public that to challenge the suggestion appears as foolhardy as arguing that the sky is not really blue. But this 'truth' is in reality a very recent phenomenon. The common belief that exercise causes weight loss can be traced to one very influential nutritionist.

French-born hero of the resistance in World War II, Jean Mayer moved to the United States just after the war. He worked at the UN Food and Agriculture Organization in Washington, DC, while earning a doctorate in Physiological Chemistry at Yale. He joined Harvard's newly founded Department of Nutrition after earning his doctorate and became a prolific and high-profile publisher of papers and books on hunger, nutrition and the then newly emerging public-health problem of obesity.

In 1959 the *New York Times* credited Mayer with destroying the theory that exercise had nothing to do with losing weight. Until the late '50s doctors had uniformly (well, as close as they ever get, anyway) believed that exercising more simply made you more hungry. Many studies had shown that patients lost more weight if they lay in bed than if they pursued vigorous exercise. It was an accepted tenet of medical practice that prescribing exercise to treat obesity was akin to prescribing beer to treat alcoholism. Banting had discovered this a century beforehand with his rowing, but it took the doctors a while to catch up.

Dr Mayer's populist writings on the subject changed all this. He published paper after paper that showed that obese people were less physically active. He drew the conclusion that being more physically active would make you less fat. His work showed definitively that fat people do exercise less than thin people, but are they fat because they exercise less, or do they exercise less because they are fat? Mayer went wholeheartedly for the first explanation and his impeccable credentials and swashbuckling war-hero charisma, coated with a liberal dash of French accent, pushed the theory into the American and then the world consciousness. Doctors didn't go down without a fight. As late as 1965, they were still writing to the *New York Times* in response to articles published by Mayer, decrying his exercise theories as nonsensical. But Mayer, like Keys, was on a mission to convince the public of his perspective, and convince them he eventually did. Ancel Keys convinced us that fat makes us fat (and gives us heart attacks) and Jean Mayer convinced us that the cure to being fat is exercise. Both managed to carry their messages in the face of strident medical opposition and both messages are core components of nutritional thinking today.

There are lots of good reasons to exercise. The Mayo Clinic says there are seven benefits to exercise. Only one of them is weight loss.

The others are improving your mood; combating heart disease by improving blood circulation; strengthening your heart and lungs; helping you get a better night's sleep; putting the spark back in your sex life; and just for fun. You could do it because it gives you an endorphin rush – that was certainly my primary motivation at university. You could do it because it gives you 'head-space'. While you exercise, your mind can wander and be free to get away from the pressures of the day. You could do it for 'you' (getting away from the kids) time. No-one is going to criticise you for devoting a half-hour to solitary exercise a day. You could do it just to feel well. There is no doubt that exercise is crucial for overall health. My point is that exercise alone won't allow you to lose significant amounts of weight, if you continue to consume large amounts of fructose.

The interesting thing that I discovered is that I felt a lot more like exercising after I lost my weight than before. When I was obese I was lethargic and apathetic. Exercise was the last thing I felt like doing. Now, I actually feel like getting out and doing something after a big meal. I'm not taking up jogging any time soon but the thought of a bit of activity no longer fills me with dread. I firmly believe that Dr Mayer chose the wrong option. Fat people do less exercise because they are fat; they are not fat because they do less exercise.

Exercise aside, the reason for the rampant explosion in mortality from diseases that nobody had heard about a century ago is, according to the experts, willpower. All of a sudden in the last 100 years of our 130 000-year history as a separate species, the human race as a whole has gone insane and lost all control over appetite. The experts tell us we are fat because we refuse to exercise enough and because we eat too much fat. Every other mammal on the planet is getting by just fine (except for the ones we adopt as pets). There are no fat lions wandering the plains of Africa. There are no obese monkeys bending tree branches in the rainforests of Indonesia. The lions are not insisting that their prey have the fat trimmed off before a meal. And neither they nor the monkeys are spotted too frequently at the gym or out for a jog. They eat when they are hungry and stop when they are full, just like our forebears did. We, the people of the twenty-first century, are the only mammals who have suddenly decided to wipe ourselves out with obesity.

We say we're trying not to be fat. Most of us are buying the 97 per cent fat-free foods. Many of us belong to at least one gym, even if we don't attend all that often. We're trying hard to cut down on fat and lower our cholesterol, but it seems that even with all that effort we are the generation that just can't stop getting fatter and sicker. Governments and medical experts, despairing at our lemming-like race towards oblivion, exhort us to stop being so lacking in will-power and take up jogging and eat more low-fat food.

We are not fat because we suddenly lack willpower or because we don't exercise enough or because we eat hamburgers at McDonald's. Of course, not exercising, or eating too much, will make us gain weight. It's a simple case of mathematics: if you consume more energy than you expend you will gain weight. We don't get fat from sitting next to fat people on the bus. We get fat from putting too much food in our mouths relative to the energy we need. That is beyond dispute. The question is why all of a sudden we want to eat more calories than we need. The diet gurus tell us that it is because we have all those shiny new fast-food restaurants tempting us from every street corner, but this is not the first time in history that there has been plenty to eat (whether it is cooked quickly or not) and modern Americans and Australians are not the first people to be exposed to a high-fat diet. Remember, the Inuit lived on nothing but whale fat for thousands of years.

Food energy is measured in calories, or kilojoules – the metric equivalent. One calorie is the same as 4.185 kilojoules (kj). Another common energy measure, although not commonly applied to people or food, is the watt. A watt measures electrical energy consumed per hour. Thinking of energy this way helped me understand what people were going on about when they talked about burning calories. At last I had something to compare it with. A 60-watt light bulb uses 60 watts of energy every hour. One watt is equivalent to almost one (0.86) food calorie per hour. The 60-watt bulb would need to 'eat' 52 calories every hour to light the room. You need about 100 calories per hour just to keep your body alive, so in light-bulb terms, an adult human is a 120-watt appliance.

The average can of soft drink contains about 150 calories. In other words, the can contains enough energy to light a room for three hours, or run a human for 90 minutes. The energy contained in petrol is also measured in calories. One litre of petrol contains about 8000 calories (about the same as a litre of olive oil), so if your car is getting 16km per litre, it is burning 500 calories every kilometre it travels.

The kill or be killed nature of evolution has ensured that a mammal that's survived as long as we have in the evolutionary chain is pretty miserly with its energy consumption. Animals that waste energy need to eat more food. Needing more food in nature

With the energy from . . .	You could . . .
One can of soft drink	Light a room for three hours
	Stay alive for 90 minutes
	Boil 2L of water
	Drive a car 250m
	Ride a bicycle 8km

Figure 10.1: We get good mileage from our food. If Detroit could manufacture a car as fuel efficient as the human body, it would get 1280km from every litre of petrol.

means more chance of missing a meal. Miss enough meals and you don't survive long enough to reproduce. Nature's a tough place and energy wasters went by the wayside many millennia ago. Our enormously efficient energy use means that all we need to travel 8km on a bicycle is the energy contained in the 10 teaspoons of sugar in that can of soft drink. To do the same thing in a car, we would need the energy contained in 1kg of sugar (200 teaspoons).

Put in this fashion, riding a bicycle 8km and not drinking a can of soft drink both have approximately the same energy effect. I know which I would rather do.

Don't consume	or	Do exercise
Can of soft drink	150 calories	Ride a bicycle 8km
Chocolate bar	294 calories	Swim laps for an hour
Fast-food burger	515 calories	Run 6km

Figure 10.2: Some actions that have equivalent energy effects.

You could work out how many calories were in a piece of food by burning it completely and measuring the heat given off. If you bothered to do that you would come to the conclusion that our food is made up of four basic components, and that each of these components has a fixed caloric value.

Fourteen per cent of our energy needs are supplied by proteins, at the rate of four calories per gram. Proteins are found in meats and some nuts and vegetables. Fifty-three per cent of our energy is supplied by carbohydrates, again at the rate of four calories per gram (carbohydrates are pretty much everything we eat that is not meat or fat). Thirty-three per cent of our energy comes from fat found in meats and vegetable oils. Fat is a more efficient energy store than protein or carbohydrate, because it doesn't need to contain water to hold it all together. One gram of fat yields almost twice as much energy (nine calories) as either protein or carbohydrate. The only other major source of energy (well, more major for some of us than others) is alcohol. One gram of alcohol stores seven calories of food energy.

Fibre is a kind of carbohydrate that we can't digest because we literally don't have the stomach for it. Cows and other grass eaters have evolved a capacity to digest fibre using an extra stomach. Since we haven't gone to so much bother, fibre doesn't yield any energy in our diet. Salads, fruits, whole grains and vegetables are high in fibre, which is why their caloric values are so low compared with their mass.

Our super food converter turns every edible part of food (which is everything except the fibre) into energy. Anything we don't immediately need for energy is stored as body fat or glycogen for later use. Our extraordinarily efficient energy use means that increasing the amount of physical exercise we do is significantly less effective at reducing fat storage than consuming less energy in the first place.

The amount of energy we need to live obviously depends on what we are doing, but an average young adult male is likely to need about 2500 calories per day, and an equivalent female probably needs about 2000 calories per day. Children, sedentary and older people require less energy and physically active people need more. If we are eating around about the average for our age and gender, around 70 per cent of the energy we consume is required just to keep us alive. This is called our base metabolic rate (BMR). An adult's brain alone consumes 25 per cent of our energy intake and a child's brain uses 45 per cent of all the energy they consume. The remainder of the BMR is used to keep our heart beating, our lungs breathing, our body temperature stable and so on. A further 10 per cent of what we eat is consumed in digesting the food and converting it to energy. That leaves us with 20 per cent for everything else, like walking to the bus, making the bed and any other exercise we choose to do. If you are an exercise nut then you will need more than that 20 per cent and you'll get it either from your stored body fat or from rewarding yourself with a can of soft drink and a chocolate bar after a workout.

When I was in university, I suffered from an extreme inability to be bothered going to lectures. Confronted with the need to satisfy people (such as my parents) who were suffering under the impression I was attending an educational institution, and having no desire to actually attend a lecture, I eventually drifted towards the very well-equipped gymnasium. The gymnasium had lots of interesting gadgets that you could use and appear to be doing something. Weightlifting in general appeared to be a form of exercise that didn't require running (not my forte – this was before everyone went treadmill crazy). Having more hours than were decent available to me, I eventually began using the equipment properly. The inevitable endorphin rush kicked in and I found myself actually addicted to working out. Spending three to four hours a day at the gym for four years had a fabulous effect on my physique. I slimmed down and was no longer the pudgy teenager who had entered that august institution. I could eat whatever I liked, knowing that I would head for the gym and burn it off. The effect lasted exactly long enough for me to fool my wife-to-be into marrying me.

As soon as I stopped exercising like a maniac, the weight I had lost (and much more) piled back on and it seemed there was nothing I could do about it. Over the years I would sporadically do a bit of exercise, but nothing ever knocked more than a kilo off and it certainly didn't seem to be worth the effort. What I didn't realise was that I had nature working against me on two fronts.

Firstly, my body was just too efficient. I had never done the maths to see exactly how much exercise was needed just to burn off that extra can of soft drink and chocolate bar I had got in the habit of gulping down, let alone actually eat into the fat stores. The reason for that was that the information isn't laid out like that anywhere. It's actually quite tricky to work through the data and come to those conclusions. But there's nothing controversial or in dispute about any of it. It's just that it seems someone forgot to publish the user guide for the human body. I can see the policy reason behind avoiding that kind of exposure. The last thing anybody in authority wants is for us all to have another reason not to exercise. But it would be handy to know anyway.

The second problem was that the kind of food I was eating was actually making it harder for me to lose weight, no matter how much exercise I did. An example probably best illustrates this. A glass of whole milk contains about 8g of fat, 8g of protein and 11g of sugar in the form of lactose. Lactose is half galactose and half glucose. Galactose is converted to glucose in the process of absorption by my body, so the carbohydrate in milk is all glucose as far as my pancreas is concerned. My hypothalamus accurately counts calories and controls the consumption of milk by monitoring the carbohydrates (using insulin and leptin), fat and protein (using CCK). My hypothalamus 'sees' every single one of the 146 calories in the glass of milk. All of the normal hormone responses are triggered and I feel appropriately full for having consumed those calories.

For decades, just about anyone in authority had been telling me that drinking whole milk was a bad thing to do because of all the saturated fat it contained. Instead, I should be drinking something much healthier like, say, a nice glass of apple juice.

A similar quantity of apple juice contains no fat (that's good, according to the health gurus – so it would no doubt be proudly labelled 100 per cent fat free), no protein, 14g of fructose, 6g of glucose and 4g of sucrose (24g of sugars in total). The 4g of sucrose is broken into its component fructose and glucose by our bodies, adding 2g each to the totals of fructose and glucose in the drink. So the drink effectively contains 16g of fructose and 8g of glucose. The glucose is counted by our pancreas just as with the milk. The 16g of fructose, however, is completely ignored by the pancreas. The fructose is converted directly to about 7g – four-ninths of 16 (the four being the calories per gram of carbohydrate, and the ninths being the calories per gram of fat) – of circulating fatty acid. This is about the same amount of fat as with the milk, but this time no CCK response is triggered because the fat was introduced through the liver, not the intestine. No glucose is created as a result of the fructose ingestion and no insulin response is stimulated.

Of the 96 calories in the juice, my hypothalamus only 'sees' the 32 calories provided by the glucose. The 64 calories provided by the fructose slips through completely undetected. To feel as full as I would after consuming the same quantity of milk, I would need to drink five times as much apple juice (about a litre). If I actually did that, I would directly create 35g of circulating fatty acids or, put another way, four times as much as I would by drinking the glass of milk. The fructose in the apple juice delivers big helpings of fatty acids while sidestepping the insulin- and CCK-driven appetite controls.

Not too many people drink a litre of apple juice in one sitting, but thanks to the marketing efforts of the fast-food and soft-drink giants, people frequently consume a large soft drink or shake with a meal. A standard large soft drink in an Australian fast-food restaurant is 600ml. That quantity of soft drink contains 68g of sugar. The sugar is half fructose. The 34g of fructose is efficiently converted to 15g of body fat and our bodies only count half the calories (139). The other 139 calories are completely ignored, giving our body permission to eat 139 more calories than we would otherwise eat in that meal. A large orange juice at the same restaurant might be smaller (only 425ml) but contains about the same amount of fructose. If you drink fructose with a meal, the fructose gives your body permission to consume many more calories without feeling full. To eat 34g of fructose in nature you would have to eat four large apples. Who could do that and still fit in a burger and fries? If you consume those fructose calories in the form of orange juice or soft drink with a meal, you will still be able to eat a large meal and not feel full, but the total number of calories you eat will be significantly higher.

All of those extra calories end up adhered to your waist and other less than desirable places. But wait, there's more. The presence of the fatty acids (created from fructose) in the bloodstream dulls the effect of insulin, eventually making us insulin resistant. This means we have to make even more insulin to respond to the calories we are detecting. Over time, as we become more and more insulin resistant, we can eat more and more without feeling full. Fructose pulls a real two-card trick on our digestive system. Its calories sneak past undetected, giving us permission to eat more. The undetected fructose gets converted directly to fatty acids and then those fatty acids degrade our ability to tell when we are full, giving us permission to eat even more.

In the 1960s, 'meal deal' packaging started to dominate the US and eventually the Australian fast-food industry. It is done to generate greater profitability by ensuring we buy a drink whether we are thirsty or not. It also ensures that when we sit down to our

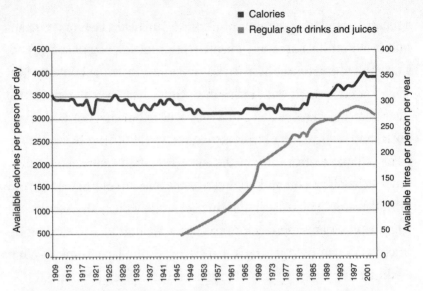

Figure 10.3: In the three decades between 1970 and 2000, the average American increased their daily calorie intake by 25 per cent and their soft-drink and juice intake by 63 per cent. In the 60 years before that, their calorie intake had barely changed at all. Notice how it takes about five years for each new peak in soft-drink consumption to flow through into increased demand for more calories. The delay is caused by fructose working its insulin resistance magic on appetite.

hamburgers and fries, the sugar in the soft drink (and the juices) permits us to eat more than we should, as well as making us fatter – I struggle to believe this is a happy coincidence for fast-food purveyors. Total calorie intake for the average American in the early 1970s was about the same as for their grandparents in 1910. However, the steadily rising wave of sugar consumption accelerated by soft drinks and juices ensured that by the turn of the twenty-first century, Americans were consuming 25 per cent more calories per day than they had been just three decades earlier. That extra 500 calories per day translates to each of them accumulating an added kilogram of body fat every two to three weeks (assuming they do nothing else to combat the weight gain). The average Australian's daily calorie intake is accelerating at a rate only slightly behind that of the average American. We are all eating hundreds of calories more per day than our parents were and then are terribly surprised when we keep getting fatter.

The average American adult consumed no added dietary fructose (besides that found in fruit) in 1850. Just 150 years later they were consuming almost 32kg per year, the equivalent of two cans of soft drink (or glasses of fruit juice) and one chocolate bar every day. The 32kg of fructose they consume every year is converted directly to 14kg of body fat and completely bypasses their appetite-control mechanism. They still eat just as much as they otherwise would, and add 14kg of body fat every year (again, assuming they do nothing else to combat it). The average Australian is not far behind, so it's no wonder that we constantly struggle to avoid gaining weight.

Exercising and dieting help us lower that weight gain but it will always be a losing battle for as long as we continue to consume fructose. To burn off that extra 14kg (and just maintain our starting weight for the year) we would need to run 7km every single day of the year (yep, even on the weekend). Staying thin in an environment where almost all food is now flavoured with fructose is like trying to row a canoe with a barbed-wire paddle. Exercise is good for you for all sorts of reasons, but losing weight shouldn't be one of the motivations. Exercising at a level that would even begin to undo the weight you put on from consuming fructose is almost impossible (if you still want to do anything else in your life). A far saner approach is simply not to consume the fructose in the first place. Fructose is a powerful catalyst for weight gain that no reasonable amount of exercise can possibly combat (unless you happen to be a bored uni student and don't care too much about CVDs, diabetes and cancer).

I lost 40kg doing no particular kind of exercise – something I am sure would dismay the producers of *The Biggest Loser*. While my way definitely makes for boring television, it's hardly surprising given how extraordinarily efficient we are at using and preserving energy. For exercise to work as claimed, we would have to be the most energy-inefficient creatures ever evolved. Exercise is certainly good for you. It keeps you toned and all your major muscle systems in good working order. We are designed to walk and run when we need to. We are, however, the only animal that feels the need to perform unnecessary exercise. We are unique in our desire to exercise purely for the purpose of losing weight. But it is a spectacularly inefficient means of achieving that goal (even if it does make for good television to watch people trying). Don't exercise if your dominant purpose is to lose weight: let a lack of fructose do that instead. If you want to go for a walk or kick a ball, then go right ahead. If you don't feel like it, then don't do it. Now, much more than I ever did before, I sometimes feel like exercising just to feel healthy or to play a sport. In fact, lethargy was one of the first things that disappeared when I stopped eating fructose.

That being said, once you do correct your appetite control by removing fructose, you will find any exercise you do feel like doing to be incrementally more effective than previously. The reason is that you will not be fighting the 'invisible' fructose calories that effectively ensured that for every step you took forward, you took two steps back. If you were previously consuming 300 calories per day in added fructose (a large juice and a couple of biscuits), then that was 300 calories your body didn't see. Those 'free' calories were directly converted to 33g of body fat, meaning you would have to swim laps for an hour every single day just *not* to gain weight. If you eliminate fructose from your diet, your body will accurately count every calorie. Any unusual exercise that you do will be financed from your fat treasury. You will feel hungry more quickly after you have done the exercise, but if you simply eat when and what you normally would, you will not eat any more than you usually do, and you will have lost the fat forever.

11. A RECIPE FOR COLD TURKEY

I am struggling to remember a day in my adult life when I didn't consider myself on a diet. Usually there was nothing formal about it. I would hear about this or that diet being raved about on the telly or mentioned in scholarly tones on the evening news, and then I would pick and choose which bits of it sounded sensible and kinda sorta be on it (or something vaguely resembling it). I would always try to buy low-fat things because everyone said you should. And in between bouts of not being able to stand the aftertaste, I would generally choose diet soft drinks. But much as dieting seems all pervasive now (just try to get through a day without seeing at least one advertisement or discussion about some kind of diet), dieting as a phenomenon is a relatively new fad. Weight Watchers, one of the first organised groups of dieters, was founded as recently as 1963, just three years before I was born. The Mediterranean diet, the first mass-market diet (invented by Dr Ancel Keys – the fat hater), was similarly only first popularised in the 1960s.

The number of overweight Americans only broke through the 40 per cent level in about 1960 (it took until 1970 in Australia). Clearly, before 40 per cent of us were overweight, there wasn't the mass-market appeal for dieting. In the four decades since the start of Weight Watchers, millions of diets have been foisted upon an eager and ever more desperate public, with no obvious benefit except to ensure that the owners of women's magazines enjoyed happy retirements. Now almost twice as many people are over-weight and cutting calories, fats, carbs, and just about everything else the fads have demanded. When my wife Lizzie announced our impending twinship, I was just as trapped in the dieting-with-no-visible-results treadmill as I had ever been. Free access to the biggest medical library in the world (the web), however, allowed me to read my way to a conclusion that, now that I see it, seems blindingly obvious. Fructose was killing me and everyone else as surely as if arsenic were being poured into the water supply.

My research had convinced me beyond all doubt that I had to stop eating fructose. I had to ensure vigilantly that as little of it crossed my lips as was possible. I had started out looking for a way not to be fat. I was now worried that being fat was the least of my concerns. I had to stop poisoning myself. If that stopped me being fat (or at least made it easier not to be) then all the better.

My first disappointment was discovering that food labellers aren't required by law to include information about whether fruc-tose is in the food we buy, and if so, how much. All the labels say is 'sugars' under the heading 'carbohydrates'. You can get massive detail on every kind of fat: saturated, monounsaturated, polyunsat-urated, trans fats (thanks, I suspect, to Dr Keys' significant influence of health policy makers). But all you get on sugars is 'sugars'. That label includes all compounds that end in 'ose', so lactose, glucose, sucrose, fructose, maltose, etc. are all lumped in together.

Take a look at a carton of whole (unflavoured) cow's milk and you will see it contains 4.7g (or 1 teaspoon) per 100ml of 'sugars'. So a litre of plain whole milk contains 10 teaspoons of sugar! But before you start tipping all your milk down the sink, it's best to remember which sugar it is – lactose. Milk does not contain any fructose, notwithstanding that its nutrition label would lead you to expect that it might contain quite a lot. There is no way to tell from the label that milk contains no fructose.

When you look at flavoured milk, it gets even more complex. A litre of chocolate milk typically contains about 100g of sugar. It's milk, so we know by a process of elimination that 47 of those grams comes from the lactose. The rest is what makes it sweet: ordinary old table sugar (sucrose). The sucrose is of course half glucose and half fructose. The litre of chocolate milk therefore contains 26.5g of fructose. It would be easier if it were just labelled that way, but I found that I got pretty efficient at doing those sorts of calculations after a while.

The good news is that we come equipped with a built-in fructose detector that allows us to sense the presence of fructose before we swallow it. I don't recommend conducting taste tests before buying (unless you fancy close contact with the constabulary), but it is a very handy way to tell whether you should be eating something. I found that I simply needed to be aware of what the detector was telling me and react in the opposite way to the way I had to date. If food tastes sweet, it probably contains fructose. The sweeter food tastes, the more fructose it probably contains. I wouldn't have known the exact numbers, but I could have detected the presence of fructose in chocolate milk by the difference in taste between it and the plain milk. My built-in fructose detector would already have told me the answer arrived at with so much label analysis and science earlier. Milk is not sweet; therefore, it doesn't contain fructose. Since any amount of added fructose is an unacceptable amount, you really don't need to do the maths.

I have never been very good at reading labels and I don't advocate it as a pastime unless you really do have nothing better to do. After several years of navigating around fructose in everyday food, I've developed some simple rules to live by. Follow these rules and I guarantee you will successfully avoid 99 per cent of the fructose in your current diet. If you follow these rules, all the weight-loss equipment you will need is already built into the body you walk around in. You will have no need of calorie-counting guides, food scales, GI tables, carb tables or fat tables. Most importantly, you will not feel like you are on a diet and after a while food tastes better anyway. This will dramatically increase your chances of sticking to this new way of eating, and it will be more likely to become simply a lifetime habit. If you achieve that, you will probably never gain weight again and you will likely have no need of any other diet again. You will disappoint millions of 'health entrepreneurs' and destroy thousands of business plans, but you will be the lean, mean machine you were designed to be from the beginning. Here are the rules:

Rule 1: Don't drink sugar

Rule 2: Don't snack on sugar

Rule 3: Party foods are for parties

Rule 4: Be careful at breakfast

Rule 5: There is no such thing as good sugar

They sound familiar, don't they? They are a lot like what every '50s and '60s mother told their children about food, but which we all seem to have forgotten (with able assistance from some pretty skilful marketing campaigns).

Rule 1: Don't drink sugar

In the modern world there are very few drinks that aren't sweetened with sugar and therefore fructose. If you are thirsty, drink water or milk. If water and milk don't appeal, you aren't really thirsty (if that doesn't sound like your mother, nothing does). All full-strength soft drinks are about 6 per cent fructose by weight. That translates to about 10g of body fat for the average 375ml can of soft drink. The most popular fruit juices are even worse than soft drink (this is probably why they are the most popular). Fruit juices often taste sweeter than soft drinks, but the fruit juice industry has very cleverly convinced us that they are, in fact, 'natural', and therefore healthy. An average apple juice is about 7 per cent fructose by weight. This means that a drink of juice the size of a soft-drink can directly creates about 12g of body fat.

These figures are for unsweetened juices – often manufacturers (particularly those targeting children) add even more sugar to overcome the tart taste of citric acid in citrus juices, or just to make it sweeter. You will be able to detect whether sugar has been added by taking a close look at the ingredients list. But at the end of the day, it doesn't really matter whether you're just drinking the fructose from the fruit or getting a little bit more from the added sugar. It's all fructose and it's all bad for you, whether it's 'natural' or added.

Ingredients: Water, mango (19%) and banana (17%) purees, cane sugar, flavour, vitamin C (ascorbic acid).

Figure 11.1: The ingredients list from a popular bottle of fruit nectar. In Australia, ingredients are listed in descending order. This 1L drink contains 132g of sugar, some of which is clearly added cane sugar.

There is a silver lining for those unimpressed by my recommendation of a water and milk fluids diet. Most alcoholic drinks do not contain significant amounts of fructose, it being one of the sugars fermented to create the alcohol. Beer contains lots of maltose but is fructose free. Most wines are largely fructose free, except for dessert wines, some sweet sparkling wines and 'coolers'. Most hard liquor is also fructose free, as long as you don't add mixers (besides water) to them. The only mixer that doesn't contain fructose is soda water (tonic water is surprisingly high in sugar). Liqueurs contain vast amounts of sugar and must be avoided. This was bad news to me; I had a bit of a coffee liqueur habit before swearing off fructose. If you can't face up to water, try switching to sparkling mineral water (without flavouring) or plain old soda water.

Diet soft drinks, of course, do not contain fructose and are perfectly acceptable substitutes as long as you are happy that the potential health effects of the substitutes are no worse for you than the fructose (see Chapter 13 on sugar substitutes). Of course, coffee and tea (being pretty much hot water with bitter flavouring) are fine to drink as long as you don't add sugar. Pre-packaged iced-tea and iced-coffee drinks are both very high in fructose.

It's important to point out that banning fruit juice doesn't mean cutting whole fruit out of your diet. Ripe fruit does contain fructose; that is, after all, where the name fructose comes from (fructus is the Latin word for fruit). A fresh apple contains about the same fructose percentage by weight as apple juice. The reality, however, is that the carbohydrate bulk and fibre contained in an apple makes it very difficult to eat the number of apples required to consume the same amount of fructose that is in the apple juice. We can all easily drink a 600ml glass of apple juice and eat a normal meal with it. Very few of us would be able to eat the equivalent four large apples and then eat a normal meal.

What's okay	What's not
Water	Flavoured waters (including children's cordials)
Coffee and tea (without sugar)	Iced tea or coffee (if they contain added sugar)
Milk	Flavoured milk
Diet soft drinks	Soft drinks
Beer, most wines and 'neat' hard liquor	Dessert wines, sweet liqueurs and alcohol with a mixer (except water or soda water)

Figure 11.2: Some common drinks and suggested fructose-free substitutes. You should really only drink to quench your thirst or get that Friday-night glow – you can still do both and be fructose free.

When fructose is consumed in whole fruit, the fructose in the fruit bypasses our appetite-control mechanisms just as effectively as the fructose in the apple juice or soft drink. What slows us down is our stomach being physically full and our digestive system having to process the 18g of fibre (60 to 70 per cent of an adult daily allowance) that the whole apple gives us. The practical reality is that most of us could not, and would not, eat more than one or two pieces (100–200g) of fruit in a sitting, and the stomach-filling effect of so doing stops us from eating 100–200g of something else as well.

Researchers now know that fibre acts to increase the effect of insulin in clearing the blood of the fatty acids created by fructose. The apple you consume still contains fructose; the difference is that there is less of it, and the damage is mainly limited to fat storage. Because of the fibre contained in the apple, you are not left with circulating fatty acids to add to your risk of a CVD, diabetes or cancer. Essentially, the fibre converts the effect of fructose to being close to the same as eating too much of anything else – it makes you fatter if you eat too much of it and don't use the energy.

Remember, our bodies have a limited capacity to process fructose and use it for energy just as if it were glucose. The fructose in those few pieces of fruit can be processed by our body. It is only when we start introducing added fructose (without fibre) that we start to cross into dangerous territory (you could call for Dr Cleave's bags of bran, I guess). If you are like most of us and fruit represents an occasional supplement rather than a large portion of your diet, then there is absolutely nothing wrong, and quite a lot right, with continuing to eat whole fruit. Just remember, fruit juice is not an acceptable substitute for whole fruit.

'Don't drink sugar' is a pretty straightforward rule. Liquid fructose delivered via juices and soft drinks is the most dangerous, simply because relatively large quantities of fructose can be ingested with no other elements (such as fibre, other carbohydrates, proteins or fat) to trigger your appetite control. Realising you need to stop drinking sugar is easy. For me, doing it was a little harder. I was on a one (at least) soft drink a day habit. If I saw a soft-drink machine outside the supermarket, I was tempted to pop a coin in the slot and get a nice cold can. I live in a tropical climate so all those pictures of ice-cold cans of drink were very tempting. The machines always sold cold water as well, but I couldn't bring myself to pay the same, or more, for so-called spring water. My preferred alcohol was gin and tonic or coffee liqueur. When I actually sat down and thought about it, cutting out fructose in drinks was going to be tricky.

The first thing I did was start buying in bulk. I would buy diet soft drinks in 24-can cartons and fill the fridge at home. This was financially as well as medically smart as they were frequently on special, which meant I was paying about a quarter as much, or even less. Whenever I felt tempted to buy a soft drink I told myself I could have one at home, and if I couldn't wait, I chose a diet version from the machine. The taste wasn't quite as good as the full-strength stuff but it still felt like I was getting a treat (which seemed to be my primary motivation). I worried a little about what the artificial sweeteners might be doing to me, but I was more worried about what I *knew* fructose was doing to me.

After a month or so, I was really getting to hate the aftertaste that comes with artificial sweeteners. Drinking soft drink was turning from a pleasurable reward into something I could easily dispense with. I decided to switch to unflavoured carbonated mineral water. It was cold, refreshing and didn't have the aftertaste, so I enjoyed it more. By then I had forgotten what the real stuff tasted like anyway, and the draw to drink it was nowhere near as strong as it had been. You might be able to go cold turkey on liquid fructose, but I needed to step down through artificial sweeteners. Since then, I haven't looked back. I found that soda water was often cheaper than mineral water so eventually I switched to that. Now I rarely drink anything other than milk or plain old tap water. No willpower is required to keep me from the sweet stuff; it just no longer appeals, and the thought of what it will do to me is enough to keep me from the remotest temptation. I still struggle to justify paying for tap water in a bottle, but if I'm out and thirsty then that's what I do.

On the alcohol front, I switched to diet tonic in my G&T and then eventually decided I preferred the taste of wine. It was much easier to switch at that level, but then again I had never been a regular drinker of anything but beer and I didn't need to change that at all. Low-carbohydrate beers have recently become popular. From a fructose perspective, the amount of carbohydrate in beer (which is maltose) is irrelevant. But if you like the taste and like paying more for beer, then go right ahead and drink low-carb beer.

Rule 2: Don't snack on sugar

It seems so harmless, doesn't it? You're standing there waiting for the jug to boil and the jar of assorted cream biscuits catches your eye. Surely just one or two won't hurt, you think to yourself. I was caught by the casual snack several times a day on just a little bit of sugar. I wasn't hungry, I just felt like a little treat. What I know now is that each cream biscuit contains about three teaspoons (14g) of sugar. Eat two of those and you are pumping 6g of undetected fatty acids directly into your arteries. Thinking about it that way helped me pause before reaching for the jar.

Unfortunately, there is no diet-drink equivalent for biscuits. They are still well and truly stuck in the low-fat ages. 'Diet biscuits' generally have even more sugar than their normal counterparts. The manufacturers have to get some taste in there somehow, and because they reduce the fat content, they compensate by loading the biscuits up with more sugar. Because I couldn't do my diet soft-drink substitution trick with biscuits, I just had to go cold turkey on them. This was probably the hardest thing I had to do in my quest to become fructose free.

Of course, just one biscuit will not do any permanent damage, but I found I needed to make a clear boundary for myself. It was much easier simply to say I was never going to have sweet biscuits at all rather than say sometimes I could and sometimes I couldn't. Whenever I did relax the rule a little, I found that by the end of the week I'd eaten a whole packet of biscuits, no problem at all. Four cream biscuits a day (two in the morning and two for afternoon tea) deliver 420 calories and 28g of fructose. This means that besides dumping 12.5g of fat into my arteries, the little snack delivers 112 invisible calories in just one day! I would have eaten 420 calories, but my hypothalamus would have counted only 308. A kilogram of body fat contains 9000 calories, so if I snacked this way for about three months, I would gain 1kg without my body ever taking account of having eaten it at all.

If I was capable of having one snack a year, then this would not have been a problem for me. The trouble was that I got in the habit of having a bikkie whenever I made a cuppa and the simple maths shows that is a short track to big problems (without even contemplating the fact that, since I lack oestrogen and wasn't eating fibre with the snack, a fair bit of that kilo of fat would still be sitting in my arteries). The thought of all this was too ugly for me, hence Rule 2: don't snack on sugar.

I did come up with an alternative that worked very well for me. I removed the jar of biscuits and replaced it with a jar of nuts: sometimes macadamias, sometimes cashews, sometimes almonds – whatever takes my fancy at the time. I can quite happily snack on the nuts instead of a biscuit. They still contain a lot of calories, but the difference is they are all being counted. If I snack heavily, I'm just plain not hungry at mealtime and either don't eat as much or don't eat at all.

The flipside to this rule is that, if you want to gain weight, you need to keep eating when you feel full. So if for whatever reason you want to gain weight, you will have to consciously resist the urge to stop eating when you feel you have had enough. For the rest of us this just means that when your body says you have had enough, stop eating, no matter how much is left on your plate or how irritating it is to throw away a half-eaten meal. The only way you would be able to get through a fructose-free 1000-calorie meal (which contains roughly two to three times the calories you need in a meal) would be actively to fight the urge to stop eating. Remember this when you are ordering and life will be less frustrating (and expensive).

	Small	Medium	Large
Burger	480	480	480
French fries	255	368	453
Soft drink	101	148	224
Total calories	836	996	1157

Figure 11.3: Calories in a typical fast-food 'meal deal'. It's surprising to many how easy it is to come by a 1000-calorie meal. A medium burger meal deal will do it.

Rule 3: Party food is for parties

Think about the kind of food you might encounter at a birthday party. A good party would have sweets, cupcakes, ice-cream, jellies, jam tarts, doughnuts, chocolates and, of course, birthday cake. Every single one of these foods is very high in fructose and should not be part of your daily diet. I wasn't in the habit of eating these foods every day (and I doubt you are either) but it is easy to slip into the habit of having ice-cream after your main meal or rewarding yourself with a few pieces of chocolate when you sit down for the evening. This rule asks you to cut out those treats.

You will notice as you go fructose free that desserts you barely noticed as sweet at all become sickeningly sweet. I couldn't find any definitive research on this adaptation of the palate to sweetness, but it definitely happened with me. It's at the point now that a plain old banana tastes almost unbearably sweet to me.

This is the rule that requires the most cooperation and understanding from your friends and family. Unless everybody you know is also going fructose free, you are going to be offered these little treats. Perhaps it's a slice of chocolate cake to celebrate a birthday at work. Perhaps it's everybody else in your house having a bowl of ice-cream after dinner. Perhaps it's attending a dinner party and being offered a dessert that your hostess spent all afternoon slaving over.

Little though they may be, it's the constant repetition of those sweet treats that does the damage. Eat just 50g (about four squares) of chocolate every night for a year and you will consume 4.4kg of fructose. That 4.4kg will translate directly to almost 2kg of extra body fat.

But sometimes you just shouldn't say no. Unless you never want to be asked to a dinner party again, I wouldn't be rejecting the dessert your friend slaved over all afternoon if I were you. This rule doesn't require you to be rude; it simply requires you to keep party foods out of your daily diet as much as you can. One thing I found helped a little is to tell people what you are doing and why. They'll usually understand and not offer you sweet food (this was especially effective for me, because everybody agreed I could stand to lose a chunk of weight and anything they could do to assist was performed at speed). I'm not saying you shouldn't eat these foods at parties, but even if you do, you're unlikely to do too much damage (unless you go to a lot more parties than I do).

Rule 4: Be careful at breakfast

One of the things that really caught me by surprise as a source of fructose was breakfast cereal. Before you snigger too much, of course I knew that the obvious ones made with things like chocolate had a ton of sugar. The ones I was surprised by were those that were heavily promoted as being healthy, high in fibre, low in fat and generally fabulous for your body. You know the type of thing – wheat flakes mixed with fibre sticks (whatever they are), some sultanas and various and sundry bits of dried fruit. I had been in the habit of eating a large bowl of a muesli-like mix of high-fibre bits and pieces with just a twinge of sweetness provided by the sultanas. I was gobsmacked to discover that my favourite healthy cereal was actually 26 per cent sugar by weight! But I needn't worry, because a little asterisk next to the sugar entry on the nutrition label informed me that it was mostly fructose (from the sultanas). That meant my average 100g bowl of healthy cereal was ladling invisible fat into my stomach at an extraordinary rate every morning. I decided to investigate the matter thoroughly and found that there were very few breakfast cereals that had less sugar than the average apple.

If you want to eliminate fructose (and I assume you wouldn't have read this far if you didn't) then breakfast is going to present the greatest challenge for you. In other meals, sweet food is generally obvious. Just don't have dessert and a sweet drink and you will have done pretty much all you need to for most meals. Skip morning and afternoon tea (at least the non-tea or -coffee part of them) and you will be almost fructose free. Breakfast is trickier because for most of us, breakfast cereals are the prepackaged, easy option and we are stuck with whatever the manufacturer chose to include. I didn't much like the look of the low-fructose options in the cereal aisle. I had eaten those wheat biscuits as a child, but usually only after adding half a cup of sugar to the mix. I did eat porridge in the winter, but only after adding honey. I decided to abandon cereal altogether and switch to toast. A few weeks without the fibre inspired me to veer towards some of the newer high-fibre multigrains. I now eat a high-fibre multigrain bread liberally smeared with Vegemite, just about the only spread without any sugar.

I realise that kind of bread is not for everyone, so I've laid out in the table on page 162 some of the other options I occasionally consider when pure wholegrain bread for breakfast gets a bit tedious. Obviously all of the figures assume that you will not be adding sugar to your cereals (or your bacon and eggs).

Does this mean you shouldn't eat breakfast cereals? Not really, as long as you are careful about which ones. Read the label. If the level of 'sugars' is less than 10g per hundred (whether they are labelled

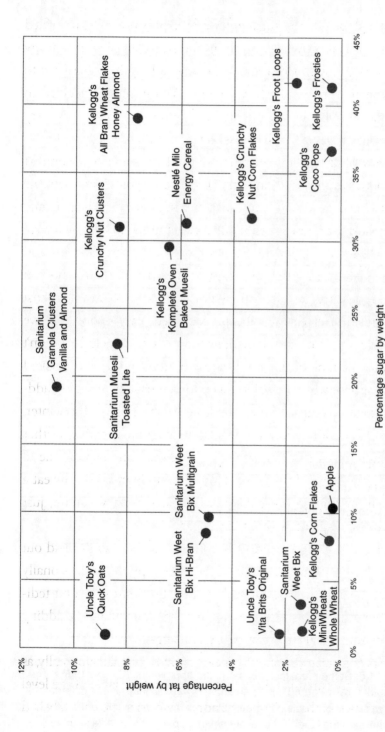

Figure 11.4: Popular Australian breakfast cereals graphed by fat (vertical) and sugar (horizontal) compared with an apple. The usual suspects are almost as high in sugar as a chocolate bar. The shock is how high some of the 'healthy' cereals are.

Food	Approximate % fructose by weight
Bacon	0%
Eggs	0%
Rolled oats	1%
Yeast extract spread	1%
Multigrain bread	1%
Pancake mix (1)	2%
Weet-Bix	2%
White bread	2%
Wholemeal bread	2%
Corn flakes	4%
Peanut butter	4%
Rice bubbles	5%
Anything below this point contains more fructose than most fruit.	
Bran flakes	7%
Raisin toast	9%
Bran sticks	10%
Fibre and fruit mix (1)	13%
Nut corn flakes	16%
High-energy cereal	16%
Sultanas and bran	17%
Sugary colourful cereal	21%
Pancake mix (2)	22%
Fibre and fruit mix (2)	23%
Maple syrup	28%
Strawberry jam	30%
Marmalade	33%
Honey	41%

Figure 11.5: Some breakfast foods and the approximate amount of fructose they contain (by weight). These percentages vary slightly across different brands of similar products. In some instances they vary significantly, so it's worth checking the label. Try to avoid anything below the middle shaded line.

as natural or not) and they also contain 2.5g per hundred or more of fibre, then they are no worse for you than eating an equivalent amount of fresh apples. Stomach distension will stop you eating too much and the neutralising effect of the fibre will stop the fructose doing too much damage. Of course you could save yourself quite a bit of money by just eating whole apples instead (a kilo of apples costs about half as much as a large box of fancy high-fibre cereal).

Rule 5: There is no such thing as good sugar

Watch out for marketing tricks. Marketers know that the smart folk among us are already wary of 'added sugar'. You've probably already noticed foods labelled 'no added sugar', a favourite among juice vendors, or 'contains only natural sugars', one the breakfast-cereal people like to use. Food manufacturers will happily tell you that because the food was already incredibly sweet, meaning they didn't have to add any sugar, it is somehow better for you. Sometimes they will say that because the food was sweetened with honey it is somehow better for you than using sugar. Strictly speaking, honey is better than cane sugar. Honey contains 40 per cent fructose compared with the 50 per cent in sugar, but neither is going to do your waistline or your arteries any favours at all.

'Natural sugar' can often be directly translated to 'contains high levels of fructose'. Fruit juices are all natural sugar – that's a huge part of their marketing message – but as we've discussed, they contain high levels of fructose. To the point that if I was dying of thirst and given a choice between a soft drink and any juice, I would have to choose the soft drink, because it probably has 10 to 20 per cent less fructose than the juice. Cereals packed with sultanas and raisins are often up to 15 per cent (26–30g of 'sugars' per 100g) fructose by weight and are full of 'natural sugar'; it's no wonder they don't need much added sugar.

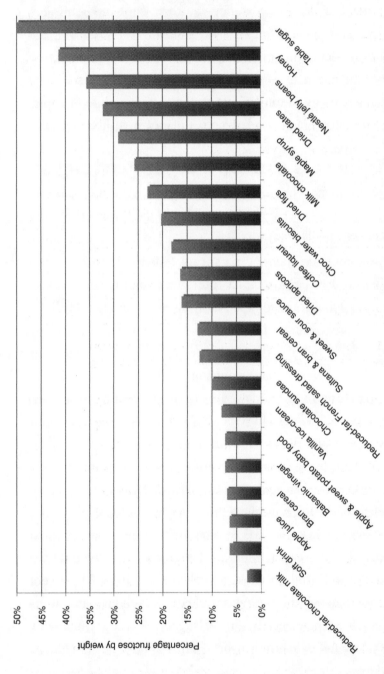

Figure 11.6: High-fructose foods (by weight). It's not all down to 'evil' processed food manufacturers. Yes, there are the expected party foods, but some of the highest-fructose products are what a marketer would call 'natural'. Take a look where honey, dates, figs and dried apricots appear. On this chart, an apple (the highest-fructose whole fruit) would appear just to the left of the reduced-fat chocolate milk.

'Reduced fat' can also often be directly translated to 'high fructose'. The food industry knows that consumers peppered with a constant barrage of 'fat is bad' messages want to see labels like this on their food. But, as mentioned earlier, the reality is that reducing fat in food recipes often means increasing sugar. Just for fun, next time you are at the supermarket compare the sugar content of a low-fat food item with its full-strength cousin. It will often contain more sugar. Here's a few to get you started:

Product	Full-fat version percentage sugar	Low-fat version percentage sugar
Peanut butter	8%	13%
Chocolate milk	10%	11%
Vanilla yoghurt	15%	17%
Vanilla ice-cream	24%	27%

Figure 11.7: Here are a few everyday examples from the supermarket shelves. Note that the low-fat version invariably contains more sugar.

I found that the fat-free labelling tactic is also a favourite with manufacturers of confectionery in particular, who frequently proclaim that their jelly sweets and marshmallows are '99 per cent fat free' or similar. That sort of advertising makes about as much sense as a soft-drink manufacturer proclaiming their products to be fat free (perhaps their focus groups told them that we wouldn't fall for that one). Sweets are almost pure sugar. The only ones that aren't are those that also include chocolate (which is one-third fat). The marketers' hope is that the '99 per cent fat free' label will convince you that you can consume foods that contain 75 per cent or more sugar without any concerns at all.

I developed a neat little rule of thumb to help me quickly tell how bad something was likely to be for me. Every 4g of sugar I saw on the label translated to about 1g of body fat (on me) that wouldn't be detected by my appetite-control system.

'Low GI' is another marketing term that I saw quite a bit of on the labels in the supermarket. As we saw in Chapter 3, a low-GI food is one that has a low glycaemic index or insulin response. The theory is that, if you eat low-GI foods, energy is released more slowly and you will not have the peaks and troughs associated with foods high in glucose. Theoretically, this means you should stay satisfied for longer and be less likely to want to eat again a short time after your last meal.

While the glycaemic index of foods is likely to be critically important in diets designed to treat insulin resistance or type II diabetes, it is very likely that it is irrelevant in the question of weight control for those of us without those conditions, since it ignores the effect of leptin in moderating medium- to long-term appetite. My experience was that most foods labelled as 'low GI' were bad for me for entirely different reasons. The GI number is prone to easy manipulation by clever marketers. Food that has a large percentage of fat usually has a lower GI rating, regardless of the amount of glucose in the product. This is also true of protein, but to a lesser extent, since proteins often end up being converted to glucose by our bodies anyway.

Since fructose is largely invisible to our pancreas it also has a low glycaemic index. You can ingest large amounts of fructose and have almost no insulin response, hence a low GI. Some low-GI foods are genuinely good for you, such as the high-fibre multigrain bread (48 out of 100) that I switched to when I found out my cereal was over one-quarter sugar. But a lot of manufacturers are using the fructose loophole to gain a marketing advantage. An obvious example of this is a hazelnut spread that is 55 per cent sugar and 30 per cent fat, but which obtains a low-GI rating (46 out of 100).

Almost any chocolate-based product will be low GI because of the high amounts of fat and fructose, but most manufacturers aren't courageous enough (yet) to label a bar of chocolate 'low GI'. I discovered that I should treat low-GI foods with extreme caution. If you're not diabetic, it is probably safer simply to disregard the low-GI label altogether and employ your built-in fructose detector. Not all low-GI food is bad, but the sweet ones most definitely are.

12. SO IS THIS A DIET?

When I started avoiding fructose I immediately started losing weight. It was almost completely effortless. Sure, initially I struggled with my soft-drink addiction and occasionally found myself taking just one (or two) biscuits when offered. But with the coping strategies laid out in the previous chapter it didn't take long before I forgot the feeling of a sugar rush. I didn't change anything else about my life. I didn't start exercising more or watching what I ate in any other way. The interesting thing was that, within a few weeks, I just wasn't that hungry anymore. I used to happily down three pieces of pizza and still want more; now I found myself eating three and having to stop because I felt painfully full. It had been a long time since I felt full like that. I was definitely eating less but it didn't require any great feat of willpower. When I did eat, I really enjoyed it. I could still eat things I loved sometimes, like pizza and sausage rolls and pies. I stopped caring about low fat. That doesn't mean I actively sought out fatty food, it just means I didn't worry about the fat content any more than I worried about the water content. I just ate whatever took my fancy. I only had one rule – no fructose. Interestingly, just as Dr Yudkin had discovered, when I told myself I could eat all the fat I wanted, I initially binged, but after a while I found myself wanting it less and less.

The weight didn't fly off – this is no bride's two-week diet. In fact, it's not a diet at all. It's just removing a single substance from the food you eat (it helped me to think of fructose like slow-acting arsenic). Rather like 'going on the bant', I lost about half a kilo a week. It took almost two years, but I lost 40kg – and then stopped. I haven't changed anything to this day, but I no longer lose weight. I still avoid fructose, but obviously my body has reached some sort of equilibrium. I don't watch what I eat. My body does it all for me. When I feel hungry I eat whatever I like (except fructose). When I am full I stop. For the first time in my life I can rely on the fact that my body knows what it is doing and trust the feedback it gives me.

If you do as I did and find your equilibrium weight is still a little higher than you would like it, and your idea of fun is not working out at the gym four hours a day, then there is one thing you might try. As I've mentioned, I found in all my trial and error that low-carbohydrate diets do actually work, so you might like to reduce your carbohydrate intake for a while. The only catch is that when you stop doing it and revert to normal carbohydrate intake, do not fall off the fructose bandwagon or you will gain back all the weight and more.

Low-carb diets are effective (at least in the short term), but if you think about it for a moment or two it will be obvious why they work initially and also why no-one can ever seem to stay on one for very long. The vast majority of our food supply is glucose (carbohydrate) based. If you decide that you will not eat most of the foods around you, you are likely to struggle to find sufficient calories in the remainder of the foods available to you. If you stick to the diet it will be a daily fight to find anything you are allowed to eat, because every vendor of food assumes that you, like the rest of us, want at least half (and preferably three-quarters) of your food to contain carbohydrates. You will likely eat fewer calories than you require out of sheer lack of choice and you will likely lose a lot of weight initially. The daily struggle to find food you are actually able to eat will eventually get to you and you will abandon the diet. Where most people go wrong is that in stopping the diet they revert to eating fructose and again mess up their appetite-control system. With no appetite control, they veer back on to the path of continuous weight gain.

Carbohydrates (except for fructose) are not bad for you. You need glucose from carbohydrates to live. If you don't get the glucose from carbohydrates, your body will switch to Plan B and get the glucose from protein, and this is how these diets work. Plan B is less energy efficient than Plan A, but okay to use in an emergency. Low-carb diets do work; they are just hard to stay with. Use them if you want to lose weight quickly or give yourself a nudge off a plateau. Don't worry too much about the details. Your body really can't tell the difference between Canadian yak butter and plain old butter. Just stop eating carbohydrates. Your body will scream that it is starving (no matter how much protein you eat) for the first 24 hours. At this point you are burning through your glycogen stores and your body is harbouring the hope that you have just forgotten to eat. After this, your carbohydrate-signalling system begins to shut down and you will no longer feel hungry. Eat proteins, salads and vegetables until you can stand it no more (I suspect about two weeks), then revert to normal. The only carbohydrate you have to avoid when eating normally is fructose, and thankfully you can rely on your perfectly functional fructose detection device. If food tastes sweet, don't eat it. If it doesn't, go right ahead – your body will tell you when to stop.

The rules I worked out to help me avoid fructose meant I could eat as much fat as my body would allow – but I do have one word of warning about that. As I read far and wide on the badness of fructose, I consistently came across studies on one type of fat that could be very bad for you – trans fat. Trans fat is a type of unsaturated fat and it, like fructose, has been added to our diets in significant quantities in the last 40 years.

Trans fatty acid molecules are made by adding hydrogen molecules to unsaturated fats like vegetable oils to make them more saturated. This gives the product a longer shelf life and a higher boiling point (which makes it good for use in frying fast food). Vast amounts of trans fats are added to our diets in this way. Margarines that have not been altered to reduce trans fats can contain up to 15 per cent trans fat (as a ratio of total fat). Vegetable oils used for deep frying in the fast-food industry can contain up to 45 per cent trans fat. A small amount of fat in nature is trans fat, too (2 to 5 per cent of animal fat is trans fat).

Trans fat looks just like normal fat to our appetite-control centres. Unlike fructose, the amount of trans fat you can consume is controlled by your appetite-control mechanisms, but it is so dangerous that even the small amount your body lets you eat should be avoided. Trans fats have a proven effect on increasing LDL (bad) cholesterol and, consequently, the risk of heart disease. So, while a fructose-free diet means you can eat as much fat as your body allows, you should avoid foods high in trans fats such as margarines and some frying oils, unless they specifically say that they have been modified to reduce trans fats. Look for labels that promote trans fats in the 2 to 5 per cent range or less on these types of foods.

Completely removing added fructose from your diet will restore your appetite to normal within weeks, if not days. Until your appetite control returns to normal (so you can tell when you are full), fruit consumption should be kept to the couple of pieces a day recommended by most nutritionists. Other than that, it is simply a case of reading labels. As a rule of thumb, you can halve the number of grams under 'sugars' per 100g for most foods to approximate the percentage of fructose in the food. You will be distressed to find that all processed foods contain some sugar, but while there is no absolutely safe level of fructose consumption, if you stay under the amount contained in a couple of pieces of fruit per day (5–10g) you will probably remain within the limits of your digestive system.

One of the best things you will find about removing fructose from your life will be that the less you have of it, the less you want it. Once your appetite-control mechanisms are working properly again, you simply won't want to eat or drink sweets or to snack between meals. You will find foods you previously ate without thought to be too sickly-sweet to enjoy. You will still reach for the chocolate, but a combination of the very sweet taste and the knowledge of exactly how many grams of body fat each piece is adding to your waistline (about 1g for every 4g of sugar on the nutrition label) will have you refusing any more than one piece (which you probably won't enjoy much anyway). People will compliment you on your admirable restraint but you will know that no great work of willpower is required; you just don't really want it anymore.

If you simply do not eat or drink food that tastes sweet you will be in 100 per cent compliance with the no-fructose rules. You can eat anything else you like (avoiding trans fats where possible), just don't eat sweet-tasting food. This rule is very hard to stick to for the first few weeks. This shouldn't come as a big surprise; you have spent your life to this point obeying your evolutionary design and seeking out sweet food. By implementing these rules you will effectively be going 'cold turkey' on sweet foods. This is the very hardest part of your new way of eating. If you can get through those initial couple of weeks, everything thereafter will be dramatically easier. But you must get through the withdrawal period. Have strength.

Once fructose is removed from your diet, you will be stopped from eating too much by your now reliable and accurate food meter. You won't feel hungry between meals and you will avoid what is probably for most of us the second-largest source of fructose in our diet, the occasional sweet between-meals snack. If you do this every day the weight will slowly and effortlessly peel away. You didn't get fat overnight and you won't lose it overnight either, but by avoiding sweet drinks and snacks you will barely notice the change in diet. Implementing the rules I've worked out through trial and error allows you to lose weight without really doing anything (except avoiding fructose). You will not feel like you are on a diet at all.

13. ALTERNATIVES TO FRUCTOSE

One of the things that made it easier for me to give up fructose was being able to switch from full-strength soft drinks to artificially sweetened ones. Thanks to the miracle of modern chemistry it was still possible to get my hit of sweetness without swallowing fructose. It seems I'm not the only one enjoying a gulp of artificially sweetened drink. Artificial sweeteners are the boom industry of the new millennium, and their existence has significantly throttled back the upward acceleration of our lust for fructose. If they didn't exist we would now be consuming almost twice as much fructose as we currently do.

There are four main artificial sweeteners. Manufacturers prefer to call them non-caloric sweeteners or high-intensity sweeteners, so as to distinguish them from other manufactured sweeteners such as table sugar and HFCS. These chemicals taste hundreds of times sweeter to us than sugar, so while they contain the same number of calories per gram as any other carbohydrate, their dieting power

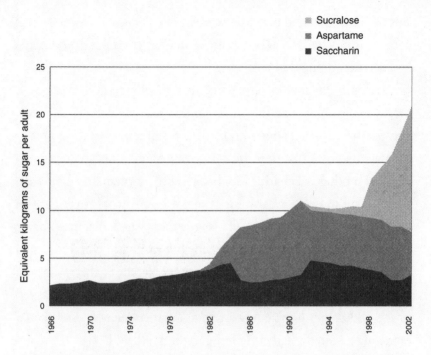

Figure 13.1: Artificial sweetener consumption has skyrocketed. The average American would be eating 21kg per annum more sugar (10.5kg more fructose) if it hadn't.

comes from the fact that much less is required to obtain the same sweet taste. For example, saccharin is 550 times sweeter than sugar, it is chemically stable when mixed with other foods and has a good shelf life. Because the human digestive system has no receptor proteins for it, it passes straight through our bodies. It therefore effectively contains no calories.

Saccharin, the oldest high-intensity sweetener, was accidentally discovered in 1878 by scientists working on coal tar derivatives at the Johns Hopkins University in the United States. Ira Remsen and his German student, Constantin Fahlberg, noticed that residue on their fingers from experiments with benzoic sulfinide tasted initially intensely sweet and then bitter. The story goes that Ira was eating a bread roll after a hard day in the lab and noticed it being very sweet.

After a bit of trial and error, he worked out that the sweet taste was coming from chemical residues on his fingers from the experiments he had been doing that morning.

Ira and Constantin wrote up their discovery in 1879, but it seems Constantin was the more commercially savvy of the two, because he arranged some funding from Germany and raced off to the patents office (much to Ira's annoyance). Constantin christened his new product saccharin, which was a little more marketable than benzoic sulfinide. It was immediately a boon in the treatment of type I diabetics (the only type of diabetic there was at that time), since they could consume foods sweetened with saccharin without raising their blood-sugar levels. This kept them safer from the ravages of (then) untreatable high blood sugar. Saccharin was commercialised in the 1880s but didn't enjoy any mass-market success until the fat epidemic inspired the dieting industry in the early 1960s.

Since 1907, there have been concerns about the safety of saccharin for human consumption. It was investigated by the USDA for causing digestive problems and was banned as a food additive just prior to World War I. During the war, a sugar shortage forced the government to lift the ban so the incessant demand for sugar could be satisfied (it would be a brave government that stood between the people and their sweet treats). Saccharin's unpleasant metallic aftertaste limited its potential market to people who really had no choice (diabetics and a country suffering from a war-induced sugar shortage).

In 1937, a partial solution was discovered. Cyclamate was also accidentally discovered in a lab looking at something else entirely. University of Illinois graduate student Michael Sveda was working on creating an anti-fever medication when he put his cigarette down on a bench where some cyclohexanesulfamic acid had been spilled. When he picked the cigarette up, he noticed a sweet taste.

Michael also raced off to the patents office to protect the discovery of what he christened cyclamate. Food additive testing was a bit tougher by then and it took a lot of money to do the necessary testing. Michael sold his patent to Abbot Laboratories, who did the testing that finally (in 1958) permitted cyclamate to be approved as safe for use in food.

Cyclamate is much less sweet than saccharin, at only 50 times as sweet as sugar. It also has an unpleasant aftertaste, but less so than saccharin and, to some extent, when they are mixed together they mask each other's aftertaste. Saccharin mixed with cyclamate (10 parts cyclamate to one part saccharin) was marketed as a sugar substitute in restaurants under the brand Sweet'N Low and was used in the first no-calorie soft drink, TAB, released by Coca-Cola in 1963.

The widespread use of saccharin mixed with cyclamate in the 1960s inspired more detailed animal studies (many funded by the sugar industry), which started to raise concerns about both chemicals possibly causing cancer. In 1969, a rat study showed conclusively that the common 10:1 mixture of cyclamate and saccharin definitively caused bladder cancer in rats. The United States immediately banned cyclamate as a food additive. In 1977, a Canadian study showed that high doses of saccharin (the equivalent of 800 cans of TAB a day) caused bladder cancer in 17 of the 200 rats in the study. The Canadian government immediately banned saccharin as a food additive. But the United States had a bigger problem: by then the US public was consuming 225 000 tonnes of saccharin (mostly in diet soft drinks) a year. When it became public that the US government was considering a ban, the howls of public protest (largely funded by the saccharin industry) were loud and long.

People didn't want to lose their diet drinks. In the end, the United States compromised by requiring products containing saccharin to carry a warning about possibly causing cancer, but a ban was not implemented. To this day, cyclamate is banned in the United States but not Canada, and saccharin is banned in Canada but not the United States. Sweet'N Low is sold on both sides of the border with different inert fillers instead of the respectively banned ingredient. Both cyclamate and saccharin are approved for use in Australia.

Cyclamate and saccharin had the market to themselves until 1981, when aspartame received US FDA approval. Aspartyl-phenylalanine-1-methyl ester, once again, was an accidental discovery. In 1965, James Schlatter, a chemist working for GD Searle & Co, was looking for an anti-ulcer drug when he licked his finger. The sugar industry ensured that some well-funded researchers lined up their rats for aspartame when its turn came to be tested. The usual doubts were raised about aspartame causing cancer, in particular brain cancer, or possibly brain damage. Many years of lobbying ensured that aspartame remained on the banned list until 1981. Soon after Ronald Reagan became the US president in 1980, GD Searle's CEO, Donald Rumsfeld (yes, that one), reapplied successfully for certification for use in dry goods. Australia quickly followed suit and approved aspartame in 1981. The US FDA commissioner who approved aspartame was Arthur Hayes. Hayes resigned from the FDA in November 1983, shortly after extending aspartame's approval for use in soft drinks, and immediately took up a position as a senior medical advisor to GD Searle's public relations firm.

Donald Rumsfeld engineered the sale of GD Searle to Monsanto in 1985. The aspartame patent expired in 1992, opening up Monsanto to significant competition. Monsanto sold the struggling aspartame business to its present owners, Merisant (a company created by Monsanto managers to buy the business), in 2000. Besides aspartame, Merisant has a substantial saccharin business branded Equal, which competes with Sweet'N Low.

Aspartame tastes similar to sugar and has the same number of calories. It is, however, 200 times sweeter, so where a soft-drink manufacturer would use 55g of sugar in a can, they can replace it (and its 220 calories) with just one-quarter of a gram of aspartame, which provides just one calorie. Unlike cyclamate and saccharin, aspartame is actually digested by the body rather than simply passing straight through. And this is the source of many of the medical concerns with it. Besides the acknowledged danger to phenylketonurics (people who suffer from a rare genetic inability to process phenylalanine – there is a warning on every product containing aspartame for these people), studies have shown all manner of adverse effects, ranging from brain tumours to brain lesions and lymphoma. Many of these studies have come in for criticism concerning their methods, motivations and results. There is big money at stake in the artificial sweetener industry and deep pockets on both sides of the argument. Rather like the controversial studies in the '60s and '70s that showed smoking caused lung cancer, there is always another study available to contradict. Two recently published large-scale studies have failed to show any adverse effects from aspartame consumed at the levels that is currently commonplace.

Aspartame is marketed as Nutrasweet and is the sweetener that I ingested large quantities of while getting unhooked from sugar soft drinks. I don't drink them anymore because after about four weeks I no longer craved sugar and I was getting sick of the metallic aftertaste of aspartame. I don't know whether it is any worse for me than fructose and I doubt anyone else does either, given it has only been commercially available for 25 years, but I took the calculated risk that a short exposure to it might not kill me. I hope I am right; only time will tell. For now, I'll stick to water and milk if I'm thirsty.

The last of the big four is sucralose. Once again the story is of accidental discovery, but this time the researchers were looking for a sweetener and they were doing it on the payroll of the biggest sugar distributor in the world, Tate and Lyle. The Tate and Lyle scientists were working with Dr Yudkin's sugar research team at Queen Elizabeth College, London, in the late '60s when they discovered that trichlorogalactosucrose (chlorinated sugar – hence the marketing spin that it is made from sugar) tasted 600 times sweeter than sugar. Sucralose is marketed as Splenda and was approved for use in food in Australia in 1993 and the United States in 1998. Like aspartame, sucralose has the same number of calories as sugar and is digested by our bodies. However, being three times as sweet as aspartame, even less of it needs to be used to obtain the same effect. Sucralose is a type of organochloride, a class of chemicals known to cause adverse effects in humans in relatively small concentrations. As a result it has undergone a barrage of testing like no other sweetener before. All approving countries have satisfied themselves that in the concentrations we are likely to consume, sucralose is safe (sounds reassuring, doesn't it?). The studies showed that when you fed mice the equivalent of 2000 cans of diet soft drink per day you could cause DNA damage. If they doubled the dose, they could cause brain damage. High doses are used in studies like this to simulate lifetime consumption quantities for us, but such an approximation is fraught with difficulties in applying the results.

One of the things I found interesting about all these rat studies was how intensively the sugar industry and its various lobby groups have targeted the task of proving artificial sweeteners are dangerous. Much more conclusive animal and human studies have shown how destructive sugar is, but there has never been a suggestion that sugar should be banned. This is not to say I am in any way reassured about the sweetener studies. Artificial sweeteners have simply not been in our diet long enough to tell. No amount of rat studies will reassure me that industrial chemicals that have been in our food supply for less than a few decades are definitely safe. Long-term trials have not been done and many in the medical community question whether they are safe for continuous human consumption. It took almost 100 years of mass consumption before researchers started questioning whether sugar was dangerous. Can we really know if sucralose or aspartame are safe after just a few decades?

Sucralose is the golden child of the $1.5 billion sweetener industry. Its sales are accelerating at an exponential pace and it now commands over 62 per cent of the artificial sweetener market. A honey pot like the artificial sweetener market is continuously attracts new players and we can expect to see a lot more chemicals approved for use in the near future. Alitame (2000 times sweeter than sugar) is already approved for use in Australia and is pending in the United States. Neotame (13 000 times sweeter than sugar) is pending approval in both the United States and Australia.

Some of the bad press about dead and deformed rats has convinced a few consumers to be wary of artificial sweeteners. Conscious of this, some manufacturers are now promoting foods as sugar free that are sweet but do not contain sugar or any of the high-intensity sweeteners. These products usually contain polyols (sugar alcohols). The more popular polyols are sorbitol, maltitol, mannitol and xylitol. Sorbitol is created from glucose. The change to the chemical structure of glucose means that sorbitol is incompletely taken up by the glucose transport proteins in our gut. As a result, a gram of sorbitol delivers only 2.6 calories, rather than the four calories contained in a gram of glucose. The other 1.4 calories per gram are ignored by our body and pass straight through. Because of this, if you eat more than about 50g of sorbitol you will experience the same symptoms as people who are lactose intolerant: diarrhoea and bloating.

Sorbitol retains the same sweetness as glucose (it's about 60 per cent as sweet as sugar), so it often needs to be mixed with a high-intensity sweetener to make it taste the same as sugar. The really bad news is that sorbitol is completely and rapidly converted to fructose by our liver. The same is true for all of the other polyols. From a metabolic perspective, eating polyol-sweetened food is exactly the same as eating sugar (except I guess slightly less of it actually gets into your system). That being the case, you might as well eat the sugar as eat food that has been altered to reduce its calories using polyols.

People worried about sugar consumption often propose honey as the natural alternative. Honey is relatively expensive, but the fact that it is natural is often promoted as giving it a halo of good-ness. Honey is 40 per cent fructose; that's why it's so sweet. From a chemical perspective, there is no practical difference between eating a teaspoon of honey and a teaspoon of sugar. Some people have said to me, 'But it's natural, so we must be evolved to deal with it.' Of course honey is natural, but it is extraordinarily difficult to get any quantity of it if you have to deal with the bees directly (try it, I dare you). Once it is farmed and conveniently placed in bottles on the supermarket shelves, it is easy to consume significantly greater quantities than you would ever encounter in nature.

The sugar industry has done its best to attack HFCS as a sweet-ener in the last few decades. HFCS has halved the value of the US sugar industry since 1980, so they have good reason to be concerned. Whispered campaigns about the evils of manufactured HFCS have raised some public doubts, but the HFCS makers have cleverly hit back with research that shows HFCS is no worse for you than sugar. In my humble opinion that's rather like saying that running someone over with a red truck is no worse than running them over with a blue truck. However, from a chemical perspective, the HFCS producers are absolutely correct. HFCS is a mix of fructose and glucose (usually 55 per cent fructose). We know that sucrose (table sugar) is a molecular bonding of fructose and glucose (50 per cent of each). As far as our body is concerned, whether they are bonded at the molecular level makes no difference; it splits them up anyway. HFCS is slightly worse for us gram for gram because it contains slightly more fructose than sugar, but manufacturers use less of it anyway, so that a product containing HFCS is no sweeter than the equivalent sugar-flavoured product. HFCS is barely used in Australia. We have way too much sugar available here to be bothered mucking about chemically altering corn syrup.

There is one substitute for sugar that no manufacturer is promoting. It isn't a manufactured industrial chemical. It tastes as sweet as sorbitol. It contains no fructose and is not converted to fructose by your liver. Your body is perfectly adapted to consume this substance without destroying your appetite system. It won't make you gain weight or give you a CVD, diabetes, cancer, tooth decay or any of the other nasty side effects of fructose (or sweetener) consumption. This miraculous sweetener is glucose. That's right, glucose, the other half of sugar. Sugar with the fructose removed.

All of the studies on sugar have consistently proved that when rats were fed just glucose, none of the ill-effects created by sugar were observed. And this is certainly logical. Your body converts all carbohydrates (except fructose) and most protein to glucose anyway.

Your appetite-control system is perfectly adapted to dealing with glucose. In fact, it has evolved on the assumption that what you eat will either be glucose or be converted to it.

When this dawned on me, I hotfooted it to the supermarket to buy a packet of pure glucose. It wasn't the easiest thing in the world to find. It wasn't in the sugar section or with the other baking items like flour and salt. Instead, I located it in the homebrew section. It's called dextrose, is sold in 1kg bags (for about $2) and apparently plays some sort of role in the construction of home-made beer. Dextrose is a little more than half as sweet as sugar and looks a little like caster sugar. I proudly returned home with my find and asked Lizzie to make a cupcake recipe substituting dextrose for sugar. The resultant cupcake is pleasant enough to eat and certainly tastes very sweet to me after a year or two without fructose, although people who are still immersed in fructose tell me it tastes bland and a little floury.

My investment in constructing a fructose-free glucose recipe has to this point been limited to the cupcakes, but having been fructose free for so long, I have limited motivation to make sweet foods at all. I think that with barely any real investment, the food industry (should it be so inclined) could easily recreate most fructose-flavoured foods using recipes that include glucose instead. If this kind of food were easily available, it would make the task of going fructose free much easier.

14. IT'S ALL ABOUT MONEY

Ask anyone in the tobacco business. An industry that exploits hard-wired evolution for profit is a licence to print money. Sugar is much better than tobacco though. Everybody consumes your product every day (not just the ones with an addiction) and you don't need to bother with all that complicated licensing and annoying problems about how and where you advertise and sell your products. And while your sugary products are costing the health systems of most nations billions of dollars, no-one is blaming (or suing) you. In fact, if the finger of blame is pointed at anyone, it is pointed at your customers for not having the willpower to resist your products.

Australia, the United Kingdom and the United States all spend more than 60 per cent of their respective health-care budgets on the treatment and 'prevention' of symptoms and diseases that the evidence shows are caused by fructose. And the demand is accelerating. The largest direct beneficiaries of this spending are the drug companies. Forty cents in every dollar spent on pharmaceuticals are for drugs used in the management of metabolic syndrome (CVDs and type II diabetes), chiefly blood pressure and cholesterol-lowering drugs, and insulin and drugs to enhance the effect of insulin. Much of the remainder relates to drugs used in the treatment of various cancers.

The drug companies donate money to the various national heart and diabetes foundations, so they can collectively continue their mission of educating the public as to the dangers of metabolic syndrome and associated symptoms and, in Australia, lobby the government for more drugs to be included in the pharmaceutical benefits scheme. We need look no further than the Australian Heart Foundation for an example of this. Its primary corporate sponsors are the major international pharmaceutical companies.

Besides picking up the tab for the health effects of sugar, the tax-payer also subsidises the production of sugar. Because it is a product that is subject to unrelenting demand regardless of the economic cycle, sugar has always been the target of government fundraising efforts. When the product is as popular as sugar, nobody knows or cares if the government takes its toll on the way through. As a result, sugar production has been subject to significant taxation and government-driven price manipulation for most of its commercial life. For centuries, sugar has been one of the world's most controlled foods. It is rationed during wars and used as a commodity to swap for foreign currency. It's also a weapon of international diplomacy and economic policymaking. Because of the politics influencing sugar, there is virtually no free trade or true market competition in the world sugar business.

The majority of nations, both importers and exporters, regulate either sugar production or consumption and price. Most sugar exporters, Australia being one of the largest, subsidise their sugar farmers and then sell sugar in the world market for less than its production cost during periods of world surpluses. The largest producer, Brazil, has very intelligently designed its economy to accommodate diversion of sugar to ethanol production (all Brazil's cars can run on ethanol or petrol) during times of depressed prices for sugar consumption and back again when prices improve.

The United States' sugar policy has been affected by statute since 1789, when the First Congress of the United States imposed a tariff upon foreign sugar. The purpose of this and later tariffs was to provide revenue for the government. Beginning in the 1970s, the energy crisis, inflation and global commodity shortages struck at the basic foundation of the US federal sugar program. The result was a dramatic increase in sugar prices and a significant decrease in the amount of sugar in the American diet. For seven years the price of sugar in the United States varied with world prices, causing chaos for US sugar planters. Furious lobbying by the sugar industry resulted in sugar being included for the first time in the US Farm Act in 1981. Subsidies were no longer paid, but price supports were reintroduced and quotas on foreign sugar were used to control supplies and support the price of sugar to producers. The combination of price supports and subsidies costs the American consumer and taxpayer roughly $3 billion every year.

The US sugar program provides a price floor, but no price ceiling, meaning the US Department of Agriculture prevents prices from falling but does not prevent prices from rising. The sugar quotas keep the price of sugar in the United States at about twice the world level. With the sugar price artificially inflated, there has been a ready market for HFCS in the United States since the reintroduction of sugar quotas in 1981. The resultant damage to sugar consumption caused by the loss of the food manufacturers, and particularly the beverage companies, has meant that sugar refining as an industry in the United States has been in unprofitable decline for the last two decades.

HFCS is manufactured by chemically converting corn syrup (almost 100 per cent glucose) into a mix of fructose and glucose. It tastes almost identical to sugar. The artificial price maintenance of sugar gave the corn producers an opportunity that they grabbed with both hands in the late '70s. Today almost half of all the corn produced in the United States ends up being turned into HFCS. All that corn largely ends up in soft drinks. HFCS is only marginally cheaper than sugar, but in an industry where billions of grams are being purchased every year, fractions of a cent per gram make big differences. The taxpayer still foots the bill.

Corn is even more heavily subsidised than sugar. The US government subsidised the corn industry to the tune of $42 billion over the five years from 1995 to 2000.

Almost all US sugar refiners have now sold up, and what remains of the industry is run largely by grower cooperatives. Big business has quit the sugar industry in the United States and is in the process of moving towards the future of US sweeteners, HFCS and low-calorie sweeteners. The US Sugar Association (a lobby group formed in 1943 to push the interests of US sugar growers and producers) is fighting hard against HFCS, sucralose and the other sweeteners, but it is a battle that it is losing on multiple fronts.

Besides sugar refiners, other casualties of the US sugar and corn programs are the people of equatorial third-world nations dependent on sugar exports to prop up their economies. Because US sugar imports have been cut by 80 per cent since 1975 as a result of subsidised sugar and corn, the economies of Central America and the Philippines have been pulverised. The US State Department estimates that reducing US sugar imports costs friendly third-world governments almost a billion dollars a year, forcing many former sugar farmers to take up more profitable export crops such as marijuana and heroin.

In Australia, we are less generous with our sugar producers and we don't have a corn industry worth propping up, but subsidies are still present. Australia's sugar industry consists of 6500 farms spread across too many electorates for the average politician to ignore. It competes in a world where just about everybody is not playing by the rules. The European Union and the United States massively underwrite their industries and this results in a market that can be dangerous territory for producers without subsidies. In 2003, the Australian government decided to give small sugar producers incentives to leave the industry so that it could be 'rationalised for long-term economic sustainability'. Almost half a billion dollars was committed to the program. It's barely a drop in the ocean compared with the billions pouring into the sugar industry in the United States and Europe, but it shows that even in Australia we are not immune from having to pay for sugar twice. First to prop up the industry that makes it, and second to fix the damage it causes.

The real winners from inflated US sugar prices are, however, the three companies that between them control 91 per cent of the market for HFCS, and their three biggest customers. The producers are Archer Daniels Midland (ADM), which controls 36 per cent of the US HFCS market; Cargill, which controls 35 per cent; and the world's largest sugar refiner, Tate and Lyle, which brings up the rear with 20 per cent through its US subsidiary, Staley. The customers are Coca-Cola, PepsiCo and Cadbury Schweppes.

Tate and Lyle operates over 65 sugar production facilities in 29 countries, predominantly in Europe, the Americas and South-East Asia. Tate and Lyle was founded in the United Kingdom in 1921 by the amalgamation of the separate refining businesses of Henry Tate and Abram Lyle. In the mid-1930s Tate and Lyle began to purchase land and set up production facilities in Jamaica, Trinidad, Belize and Mauritius. In 1965, Tate and Lyle diversified into agribusiness and chemical research, leaving fewer resources to improve sugar technology or yields. In the mid-1970s Tate and Lyle sold its plantations and began to concentrate on importing and refining in the United Kingdom. This left countries that produce and sell raw sugar with the most risky part of the business.

In 1985, Tate and Lyle took a significant stake in the US sugar-beet-refining market, buying eight refineries operating under the name Western Sugar. A year later Tate and Lyle tried to buy into the UK beet-processing market. The British Monopolies and Mergers Commission vetoed this acquisition because it would have given Tate and Lyle control over 94 per cent of the British sugar market.

In 1988 Tate and Lyle made an ill-fated move to consolidate the fragmented US sugar-refining market, purchasing Amstar (a cane refiner using the brand name Domino Sugar) and Staley Continental (a producer of HFCS). In the late 1990s, Tate and Lyle, in response to the volatile sugar market in the United States, began seeking a buyer for its sugar holdings. In 2001, Tate and Lyle sold the Domino Sugar brand to the Sugar Cane Growers Cooperative of Florida and the Florida Crystals Corp. A year later, over 1000 sugar beet growers in Colorado, Nebraska, Wyoming and Montana united to form the Western Sugar Cooperative and purchase Tate and Lyle's remaining US sugar-refining interests. Prior to the sale, Tate and Lyle accounted for more than 20 per cent of the US sugar market.

Tate and Lyle is still the king of the world sugar industry, but much like an oil company investing in solar energy, it is making sure it has its fingers in the alternative pies as well. Tate and Lyle is the owner of the sucralose patent (developed all those years ago with the help of the Queens College team investigating the evils of sugar). Sucralose is the runaway train of the alternative sweetener market and I wouldn't mind betting that Tate and Lyle are ensuring they are well positioned if the world suddenly decides sugar is too dangerous.

ADM and Cargill are as US home-grown as they get. Both can trace their roots to the linseed-crushing industries that flourished in the US Midwest from the 1870s to the 1920s. Linseed was crushed to produce linseed oil, a polyunsaturated oil suitable for use in oil paint, a slow-drying, hard-wearing external paint that was perfect for the rapidly expanding settlements of the United States. But by the 1940s oil of a different kind was making the linseed oil business look decidedly ordinary.

Black gold, Texas tea, was cheaper and easier to use than linseed oil. The lack of interest in linseed oil (it was to be several decades before Dr Keys got everyone all hot and bothered about eating poly-unsaturated oils rather than mixing them with paint) forced ADM and Cargill to diversify into corn and soy. As it turns out, corn and soy were exactly the right things to be growing when Europe ran out of food at the end of World War II. ADM and Cargill made a killing exporting heavily subsidised US grains as part of the effort to rebuild Europe. Both companies ended up in the HFCS business as a direct extension of their grain businesses. Today they are heavily diversified commodity houses, but each controls one-third of the US HFCS business, which is worth about a quarter of a billion dollars in profit to each of them every year, most of it as a direct result of government subsidisation.

Sixty per cent of the output from all those sugar growers, corn growers, multinational sugar corporations and grain buyers ends up in the carbonated soft drinks made by just three companies, Coca-Cola and PepsiCo in the United States and Cadbury Schweppes in the United Kingdom. But these three don't just sell carbonated soft drinks. All have diversified into 'sports' drinks and juices as well. They are not the only suppliers of fructose in the world, but together they account for a significant and growing slice of the market. In 2006, PepsiCo made a profit of almost $2.5 billion, and Cadbury

Schweppes, $3 billion. Both were a mere shadow of Coca-Cola's almost $11 billion. Together, these three chalked up $16.5 billion in profit – about the same as the big two of the tobacco industry, Altria (Phillip Morris) and British American Tobacco – on sales of over $100 billion, and it was just an average year in the soft-drink game. There's nothing wrong with being in the business of selling products that every human on the planet is hardwired to consume. The difference between sugar and tobacco is that the sugar industry has us all convinced it is our fault we're fat, not theirs.

Another sector that benefits from the mass self-delusion that we are to blame for being fat is the dieting industry. Going to the gym is a popular 'cure'. People in the United States spent $21 billion doing that in 2006. They also spent $20 billion on diet soft drinks, $4 billion on meal replacements, $3 billion on low-calorie meals, $3 billion on pharmacy diet programs, $2.5 billion on artificial sweeteners, $2 billion on diet books, $2 billion on weight-loss centres and a mere $1 billion on anti-obesity drugs. The total US weight-loss industry is worth over $58 billion a year and is growing at about the same rate as our waistlines (6 per cent per annum).

Chaos theory is infamously misquoted as saying that a hurricane in the United States can be caused by the flap of a butterfly's wings in Tokyo. Fructose is the mother of all butterfly-wing flaps. A small metabolic difference in the way our bodies process fructose versus glucose has resulted in a large percentage of the human race developing varying stages of metabolic syndrome. Consumers spend billions buying the stuff, governments spend billions ensuring that consumers can continue to buy it and then hundreds of billions 'treating' the health problems created by it. And all the while, we all keep getting fatter and sicker, apparently because we lack the willpower of our grandparents.

If a nanoportion of the money spent on any one of the consequences of fructose were instead directed towards removing fructose from our diet, the world would be a significantly healthier place – and we'd stop having to listen to those endless government commercials beseeching us to show restraint and go to the gym for God's sake. Sure, some very big companies would have to find something else to do with their time, but they are full of smart people; I'm sure they can figure out something to do.

Fat in our arteries kills us. We are designed not to eat too much fat. We are also designed to seek out sweet food because it shouldn't kill us. Fructose, the substance that makes food sweet, does not occur in significant quantities in nature. But we were smart enough to figure that out and extract the fructose. When we concentrate fructose so we can make everything sweet, we open up a loophole in our body's evolved assumptions about what we will be eating. Fructose is converted to fat, but there is no control in place to stop us eating too much of it. Now the fat that we would normally eat fills our arteries, plus the fat converted from fructose. Worse than that, the fructose ruins our ability to tell when we are full.

My generation (I was born in 1966) is the first to receive an infusion of fructose every day of their lives. The results are in. If you feed humans fructose for the first 40 years of their lives you get an obesity epidemic, and massive health system costs associated with treating cardiovascular disease, type II diabetes, oral health, cancer and miscellaneous other problems. It's time to stop. You can stop eating fructose by using the fructose detector in your mouth. An even better solution would be for those who produce food to use glucose instead.

Selling fructose makes you rich, so there are many very well-heeled groups and corporations who will not like the message in this book, and I expect the attacks will come from all quarters. But we now know enough about the chemistry of the human body to be absolutely certain that fructose is a killer of epidemic proportions, and any amount of muddying of the waters by the vested interests should be treated in very much the same way as those in the tobacco industry were. Let the food fight begin!

NOTES

1. Starting out

The Saccharine Disease by T. L. Cleave (John Wright & Sons, Bristol, 1974) is usually available secondhand from Amazon.com for under $50.

A few of the sites I found particularly useful when searching for trusted articles on medical mumbo jumbo were:

- www.medbio.info, a site that I was too ignorant to understand when I started out, but later discovered to be a goldmine of relevant information. Over and over again I found the summaries and references on this site to be invaluable kicking-off points for further research. The site is authored (without any real fanfare) by Professor Emeritus Robert Horn from the Institute of Medical Biochemistry, University of Oslo, Norway.

- www.pubmedcentral.nih.gov, a massive online library of articles covering the life sciences and biochemistry. PMC is managed by the US National Institute of Health's National Center for Biotechnology Information (NCBI) in the National Library of Medicine. It is as comprehensive as it is authoritative and, best of all, it is *free*. There are a lot of online libraries that will let you access journal articles for a fee, but few can match the coverage of PMC.

■ http://jn.nutrition.org, an extensive online library of articles which appear in the *Journal of Nutrition*, published by the American Society of Nutrition (www.nutrition.org). Not all the articles are free but significant numbers are, and it is a very decent resource in the area of nutrition research.

■ www.wikipedia.org, an invaluable resource. Don't worry, I didn't take it as gospel on medical research, although I discovered it was right more often than not (the trick is picking when it's wrong). Where it came in terribly handy was in providing me with a layperson's definitions of words that medical researchers threw about with no explanation whatsoever.

Throughout the book I have used 5g as an approximation for the amount of table sugar in a teaspoon. Purists will know that it's actually 4.2g, but using that figure just makes the calculations messier without adding a greater degree of clarity to the story.

The figures on lactose intolerance rates come from an article on eMedicine.com (www.emedicine.com/med/topic3429.htm), with some cross-referencing for Australia to an article by Davidson, G.P. 1984, 'Lactase deficiency diagnosis and management', *Medical Journal of Australia*, Sept 29, pp. 442–4. In Australia, the figure of 70 per cent is more than reversed, with only 10 per cent of the adult population experiencing lactose intolerance. This will change into the future as more and more of our immigrant population comes from a non-European background.

2. Theories of fatness

You can read the 'official' version of the life and times of Dr Atkins at his company website www.atkins.com.

William Banting's book, *A Letter on Corpulence* (Harrison, 1863), is available in full online at www.lowcarb.ca/corpulence/, but be warned: it isn't exactly easy reading. This from the introduction:

'Of all the parasites that affect humanity I do not know of, nor can I imagine, any more distressing than that of Obesity, and, having emerged from a very long probation in this affliction, I am desirous of circulating my humble knowledge and experience for the benefit of other sufferers, with an earnest hope that it may lead to the same comfort and happiness I now feel under the extraordinary change,—which might almost be termed miraculous had it not been accomplished by the most simple common-sense means.'

Dr Stillman's first book, *The Doctor's Quick Weight Loss Diet*, first published in 1967 by Prentice Hall, has been republished as recently as 1987 (by Dell). You'll struggle to find it new anywhere, but there are usually secondhand copies available on Amazon. He followed this book up with *The Doctor's Quick Inches Off Diet* (Prentice Hall) in 1969, *The Doctor's Quick Teen-Age Diet* in 1971 and his *14 Day Shape-Up Program* (Delacorte Press) in 1974.

Dr Atkins' Diet Revolution (Bantam) was first published in 1972. It was republished by Avon in 1992 as *Dr Atkins' New Diet Revolution* and is still in print today. You should be able to obtain a copy of it from your local bookstore.

The most recent and outrageously popular Australian version of the low-carb diet is *The CSIRO Total Wellbeing Diet*, published in 2005 by the good folks who brought you this book and available at all good bookshops (hopefully my cheque is in the mail).

3. How we turn food into energy

If you want to read about Dr Frederick Banting (no relation to our fat friend, but an extraordinary coincidence) and Professor John MacLeod and the story of how insulin was discovered as a treatment for diabetes, go to the Nobel Prize website at http://nobelprize.org/nobel_prizes/ medicine/laureates/1923/. You can read their acceptance speeches, see photos of them and drill into the detail of why the prize was awarded to them. This site is a great resource for information on each of the numerous Nobel Prize winners that I discuss from this point on.

The graph comparing high-GI and low-GI foods has been reproduced from the Wikipedia commons. It was prepared by Studio34 in August 2006.

Dr Jennie Brand-Miller's *GI Factor: The Glucose Revolution* (Hodder Headline, 2002) was the first in a series of books she published about GI, including recipe books, kids' books, reference books and more books on how GI is used. Most of these books are still available today from your local bookshop.

4. Using stored energy

If you really like reading about the detail of some of the early discoveries in endocrinology such as Banting (from the last chapter) and Murlin, then it might be worth picking up a copy of Victor Cornelius Medvei's *The History of Clinical Endocrinology: A Comprehensive Account of Endocrinology from Earliest Times to the Present Day*, (Pantheon, 1993). It's unfortunately not easy to come by and a library might be your best bet. It's not as dry as it sounds, really.

Kojima and Kangawa's paper on the discovery of ghrelin is available in full online at http://physrev.physiology.org/cgi/content/ full/85/2/495, but I don't recommend reading it unless you are well on your way to completing your biochemistry studies. They say they named ghrelin 'after a word root ("ghre") in Proto-Indo-European languages meaning "grow"'. I still reckon they named it the way I suggest in the text and sought out an academic explanation for it, but you be the judge.

5. Fat makes you fat ... or does it?

For those who don't indulge in 'reality' television, *The Biggest Loser* is a long-running show that squeezes hundreds of hours of entertainment out of torturing a brigade of heavily obese individuals with extreme exercise routines (and some mind games for fun).

The graph showing fat consumed was prepared by me using data from the US Department of Agriculture (USDA). The USDA's Economic Research Service maintains an extraordinarily detailed open-access dataset on consumption of most foods and food groups in the United States (many, such as fats, going back to 1909). This excellent resource is located at www.ers.usda.gov/data/FoodConsumption/.

An excellent summary of the Seven Countries Study is available on the University of Minnesota Website at www.epi.umn.edu/research/7countries/overview.shtm.

Ancel Keys and his wife Margaret first published their Mediterranean Diet in 1959. The book was called *Eat Well and Stay Well* and was published by Doubleday. It's out of print now but you can usually get a second-hand copy on Amazon.

If your subscription to the *American Journal of Epidemiology* is up to date, you will find a copy of Dr Mann's Maasai study in Volume 95 on page 26. For the rest of us, a free abstract is available at http://aje.oxfordjournals.org/cgi/content/abstract/95/1/26.

Dr Yudkin's first book, *Sweet and Dangerous: The New Facts About the Sugar You Eat as a Cause of Heart Disease, Diabetes, and Other Killers*, David McKay Co, 1972, is an excellent read, if for no other reason than to get detailed insight into the earliest experiments on intentionally feeding animals sugar and measuring the results. Like just about everything else I recommend you read, it is out of print, but can still be obtained easily on Amazon.

The American Diabetic Association's 2002 directive to avoid fructose is contained in the report entitled 'Evidence-based nutrition principles and recommendations for the treatment and prevention of diabetes and related complications', which can be found online at http://care.diabetesjournals.org/cgi/content/full/26/suppl_1/s51. Strangely, the 1984 recommendation that people should eat fructose is not online anywhere.

6. Biochemistry 101

Almost nobody bothers to explain any of the basic terminology or concepts when they write biochemistry papers for publication. Something that helped me enormously in coming to grips with this stuff was a book my father-in-law Dr Tony Morton (see acknowledgements) gave me. I heartily recommend you obtain a copy of *Harper's Illustrated Biochemistry* (McGraw Hill) if you want to drill any further into the complex world of the biochemist. I use the 2006 edition, but I'm sure you'll be able to pick up a later edition at your local university library. The 2006 edition doesn't have much coverage of fructose, but it does provide a foundation to the concepts discussed in this chapter. Keep it by your side when reading biochemistry papers you discover on the internet. You'll need it, or something like it.

7. Honey without bees

The sweetness receptor gene in humans was first identified in research published by the Howard Hughes Medical Institute in 2001 (Nelson, G, Hoon, M, Chandrashekar, J, Zhang, Y, Ryba, N & Zuker, C, 'Mammalian Sweet Taste Receptors', *Cell*, vol. 106, Issue 3, pp. 381–90, online at www.cell.com/content/article/abstract?uid=PIIS0092867401004512). Follow-up research in 2005 suggests that domestic cats (being carnivores) have not evolved the gene and therefore are not attracted to sweet food. You can read the published cat research at www.plosgenetics.org/article/info:doi/10.1371/journal.pgen.0010003.

The USDA's Agricultural Research Service (yep, the people who run Beltsville) maintains a fabulous online database of the nutrient contents of over 7500 foods. You can access it at www.ars.usda.gov/main/site_main.htm?modecode=12354500.

We don't have anything equivalent to the public version of the USDA databases in Australia, but if you want to do a bit of analysis you can pull together data on what Australians eat from the National Nutrition Survey (NNS) and the National Health Survey (NHS). The NNS was a one-off, but the NHS is conducted every three years by the Australian Bureau of Statistics. Both are available from www.abs.gov.au/.

The price of sugar through the centuries is extracted from Noel Deer's 1949 two-volume epic, *The History of Sugar* (Chapman & Hall). His prices have been fed through an inflation calculator and currency converter to present them in 2007 Australian dollars. Obviously they are, at best, guesses, but they give a relative feel for the cost of white gold through the ages. Noel points out that sugar in 1400s England was almost seven times as expensive as honey (which wasn't all that cheap to begin with).

I created the graph of fructose consumption before I wrote even a word of this book. It was extraordinarily difficult to gather together all the information required. It existed, but not in any one place. The data from 1909 onwards was pulled from the USDA databases, one foodstuff at a time, by breaking out the percentage of the food (e.g. sugar, 50 per cent) that was fructose for each year and then totalling it. The figures prior to 1909 came from the *Union Army Data Set*. This incredible resource crossmatches the medical records of more than 35 000 men mustered into the Union Army with the US census results from 1850 to 1910. It provides quite an accurate representation of sugar consumption in the United States at that time, as well as lots of other interesting stuff about soldiers' socioeconomic circumstances and health. It's freely available at the University of Chicago's Center for Population Economics website: www.cpe.uchicago.edu/unionarmy/unionarmy.html.

8. Porridge in the arteries

The BMI calculator has been reproduced from the Wikipedia commons. It was prepared by InvictaHOG in September 2006 and is based on World Health Organization data, which can be viewed at www.who.int/bmi/index.jsp?introPage=intro_3.html. That WHO site is a fascinating resource. It allows you to do graphical and map-based comparisons of BMI data between countries and over time for most of the world. Take a look, it's worth it.

The US overweight and obesity graph was created by me based on data from the US Centers for Disease Control's National Center for Health Statistics (CDC-NCHS). If you want to drill down further on US health statistics, take a look at their site at www.cdc.gov/nchs/. There is an equivalent site maintained by the Australian government. The Australian Institute of Health and Welfare's site is located at www.aihw.gov.au/. Most of the statistics on disease prevalence and incidence in this and the following chapters come from one or other of these two sites.

9. More killers

The World Health Organization maintains quite thorough worldwide data on the prevalence of diabetes. You can check out their latest data and, more importantly, their predications at www.who.int/diabetes/facts/world_figures/en/.

The lung cancer versus smoking graph was created using lung cancer death rates from the CDC-NCHS and the US Mortality Volumes; you can access this at www.cdc.gov/nchs/datawh/statab/unpubd/mortabs/hist-tabs.htm. That data was combined with USDA cigarette-consumption data to produce the graph.

The graph comparing fructose consumption and prostate cancer death is not prepared using sophisticated medical statistic models. When I looked at the fructose consumption statistics, I just noticed that the curve looked similar to that of the prostate cancer data (from the mortality data referred to earlier), and fashioned a prediction by simply copying the rest of the fructose curve and attaching it to the end of the prostate cancer curve. The maths might not be there, but it looks pretty convincing to my untrained eye.

The Nurses' Health Study has been used to study just about every disease affecting women in the United States since 1976. You can read more about it at www.channing.harvard.edu/nhs/.

10. What about exercise?

Food energy is measured in calories. One calorie is the amount of energy required to increase the temperature of 1g of water by one degree centigrade. To heat enough water for a cup of coffee from room temperature to boiling point would take about 20 000 calories of energy. A calorie is a very small unit of measurement, so dieticians often abbreviate kilocalories (thousands of calories) to 'Calories' (capital 'C') as a sort of shorthand. Heating the cup of coffee would actually take just 20 Calories in the sense most people understand, as used in food labelling. The metric equivalent of the calorie is a joule, and is calculated using Einstein's famous equation $E=mc^2$, where E is energy in joules, m is mass in kilograms and c is the speed of light in metres per second. One calorie (small 'c') is equivalent to 4.185 joules and one Calorie (capital 'C') is the same as 4.185 kilojoules (kj). I've used Calorie throughout the book in lower case, where one calorie equals 4.185 kilojoules.

Jean Mayer was responsible for much more than convincing us all that exercise caused weight loss. For a full run-down on his achievements, take a look at his obituary in the *New York Times*, which you can look up in their archive at www.nytimes.com. The Mayo Clinic's summary of the seven benefits of exercise can be found at www.mayoclinic.com/health/exercise/HQ01676.

Unlike many in the fast-food industry, McDonald's publishes comprehensive nutrition data on every type of food they sell. You can download the complete dataset from the McDonald's Australia website at www.mcdonalds.com.au/HTML/nutrition/.

The graph comparing calorie intake and soft-drink consumption was created using data from the USDA's Economic Research Service online database mentioned previously.

11. A recipe for cold turkey

What is supposed to be on a food label in Australia is determined by Food Standards Australia and New Zealand. Their website at www.foodstandards.gov.au/ contains a mine of information.

The breakfast cereal graph was created by wandering the aisles of the local supermarket and jotting down the sugar and fat content of every cereal I could find. Yes, I did look seriously weird doing that, but it is the only way to find this stuff out in any sort of methodical fashion.

Whenever you see me give a number for the percentage of fructose in a vegetable or fruit, it is an average. The actual amount will depend on the variety, where it was grown, how ripe it is and, of course, the size. I've tried to be very fair and choose middling numbers for dry uncooked fruit and vegetables in all instances.

12. So is this a diet?

For a comprehensive summary of current information on trans fats, you could do worse than the American Heart Association website. I don't agree with much that the AHA says about fat, but this is worth a look: www.americanheart.org/presenter.jhtml?identifier=3045792.

13. Alternatives to fructose

The graph on artificial sweetener consumption is created from data published by the USDA Economic Research Service.

14. It's all about money

Data on the Australian sugar industry comes from www.canegrowers.com.au, a lobby group for Australian sugar-cane growers. Don't worry, I crosschecked with data from the Australian Bureau of Statistics where it was available.

Information about each of the companies discussed in this chapter was gathered from their respective corporate websites and annual reports.

ACKNOWLEDGEMENTS

Many people helped me to write this book. Some of them intended to, but for quite a few it was the last thing on their mind. Some members of the medical fraternity (who probably last looked at a biochemistry textbook sometime before Princess Di's wedding) found the fructose theory quite amusing. Their doubt forced me to make sure I understood the current research at the deepest possible level.

Lizzie tired very quickly of my regaling everyone I met with the latest article on the chemical interactions of the GLUT transports, and politely suggested that perhaps I could write a book about it. Judith (a published author) had the misfortune to sit next to me at a business breakfast. The horrors of fructose ruined her meal, but her encouragement put me on the path to writing this book.

Lizzie supported me without question (and with considerable patience) through all my strange experiments with food and convoluted explanations. She denies harbouring a hope that if I wrote it down I would shut up about it. But if that was her plan, it backfired badly when Frank (my good friend and 'agent') convinced Julie and Ingrid from Penguin that my thoughts were worth inflicting on more than those within hearing distance.

The only person who has read every draft of this book since it was 10 pages long, and fastidiously corrected (almost) all the split infinitives along the way, is my father-in-law, Dr Tony Morton RFD, MBBS, MS, MD, MScAppl, FANZCA (retired). He hates any big show being made of his qualifications, but it gave me enormous comfort to know that someone with as impressive a list as that was looking over my shoulder. Tony wrote a book on medical statistics in his retirement (just for fun), so he was a good person to make sure I didn't get too crazy with the conclusions I was drawing or the sources I was using.

Sharon and Gordon (also a doctor) have shown a level of interest and support normally reserved for fanatical adherents of cult religions. That, combined with their lifelong ability to be just ahead of the trend curve in everything from cars to music, gives me hope that this book will start the revolution we need to have in understanding obesity.

I'm still not sure if the only doctor I know who is actually an endocrinologist entirely believes everything I say about fructose. But at least Adam is no longer pointing and laughing. His early warning that I should stick to well-regarded journals stood me in very good stead.

Brooke had the unenviable job of knocking all the rough edges off my manuscript (and making me think I wrote it that way in the first place). And just when I thought it was looking pretty good, along came Jane and triple-checked everything again. I tend not to be detail oriented when it comes to finishing things I start, so having Brooke and Jane drag me that last mile was invaluable indeed. Any mistake that escaped the Penguin editorial process well and truly deserves its freedom.